Advances in
Clinical
Andrology

Advances in Clinical Andrology

Edited by

C.L.R. Barratt and I.D. Cooke

Harris Birthright Research Centre for Reproductive Medicine
Department of Obstetrics & Gynaecology
University of Sheffield
Jessop Hospital for Women
Sheffield

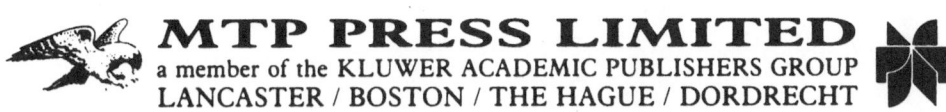

MTP PRESS LIMITED
a member of the KLUWER ACADEMIC PUBLISHERS GROUP
LANCASTER / BOSTON / THE HAGUE / DORDRECHT

Published in the UK and Europe by
MTP Press Limited
Falcon House
Lancaster, England

British Library Cataloguing in Publication Data

Advances in clinical andrology.
1. Andrology
I.   Barratt, C.L.R.   II.   Cooke, I.D.
616.6

ISBN-13: 978-94-010-7048-5   e-ISBN-13: 978-94-009-1237-3
DOI: 10.1007/978-94-009-1237-3

Published in the USA by
MTP Press
A division of Kluwer Academic Publishers
101 Philip Drive
Norwell, MA 02061, USA

CONTENTS

FOREWORD

Infertility is a problem for the couple and evaluation of the couple is preferable in a clinic where both males and females may be seen together. The contribution to care by the urologist and the gynaecologist each with an interest in infertility is different but complementary. My appreciation of this was sharpened between 1976 and 1985 during my association with the World Health Organization's Special Programme of Research Development and Research Training in Human Reproduction at the meetings of the Steering Committee of its Task Force on Infertility. The deliberations of this group were aimed at developing a protocol for investigation of the infertile couple and it became apparent to me as a gynaecologist how important is the precise characterization of the male partner's role to the formulation of the management plan for the infertile couple.

To improve the quality of our evaluation of the male partner our technical staff were trained in the semen methodology of the laboratory of Dr F Comhaire of Ghent and we were joined by Dr CLR Barratt, male reproductive biologist. It seemed appropriate to share our enthusiasm for clinical andrology, so after discussion with Dr Comhaire and Professor T Glover, an eminent male reproductive biologist, then of Brisbane, who planned a sabbatical to his native Yorkshire, a meeting was arranged for 1 and 2 May 1986. Professor Glover encouraged us to produce a small work encapsulating the details of the meeting. Although the practical sessions could not be reproduced, Dr Barratt has liaised with the speakers to produce this volume; the questions and answers at the end of each session have been retained.

The objective of the volume is to provide a current view of a number of important areas in the assessment of male infertility that will dovetail with an equally comprehensive evaluation of the female so that standards will improve for the benefit of the couple. It is addressed to all those who are interested in male infertility, either those who evaluate the males themselves or those who interpret the results of others' assessments.

Miss Anne Jequier describes a basic review of history and physical examination. Computerization of these data and considerations of the natural history of infertility are presented by Dr Frank Comhaire and his colleagues. Professor Tim Glover evaluates the difficulties in semen analysis. Dr Comhaire goes on to explore the role and treatment of the varicocele and other methods of treatment. Mr W F Hendry describes the role of the urological surgeon in evaluating azoospermia and the clinical and laboratory assessment of immunological causes of male infertility. In support Dr Adeghe and his colleagues dissect the current methods for evaluation of immunological problems. Dr Chris

Barratt describes the difficulties in evaluating infection of the male accessory glands and Dr John Aitken explores the potential of new tests of sperm function particularly sperm oocyte interaction. All authors have contributed excellent chapters in controversial areas.

It is hoped that this small book updated and extended after the meeting will be as stimulating to its readers as the original meeting was to its participants.

Professor I.D.Cooke

LIST OF CONTRIBUTORS

JH Adeghe
Department of Obstetrics & Gynaecology
Queen Elizabeth Medical Centre
Edgbaston
Birmingham B15 2TT

RJ Aitken
MRC Unit of Reproductive Biology
37 Chalmers Street
Edinburgh EH3 9EW

JS Clarkson
MRC Unit of Reproductive Biology
37 Chalmers Street
Edinburgh EH3 9EW

FM Comhaire
Department of Internal Medicine
Endocrinology Unit
State University Hospital
De Pintelaan 185
B-9000 Belgium

J Cohen
Department of Zoology Comparative
Physiology
University of Birmingham
Birmingham B15 2TT

TT Farley
World Health Organization
Special Programme of Research
Development and Research Training in
Human Reproduction
1211 Geneva 27
Switzerland

TD Glover
Department of Animal Sciences and
Production
University of Queensland
S Lucia
Brisbane
Queensland 4067
Australia

WF Hendry
Department of Urology
St Bartholomews Hospital
London EC1

DS Irvine
MRC Unit of Reproductive Biology
37 Chalmers Street
Edinburgh EH3 9EW

AM Jequier
Department of Obstetrics Gynaecology
University Hospital
Queens Medical Centre
Nottingham NG7 2UH

DW Richardson
MRC Unit of Reproductive Biology
37 Chalmers Street
Edinburgh EH3 9EW

E Rombaut
AKB Medical Ltd
Charles De Kerckhovelaan 359
B-9000 Ghent
Belgium

PJ Rowe
World Health Organization
Special Programme of Research
Development and Research Training in
Human Reproduction
1211 Geneva 27
Switzerland

FA Schoojans
Department of Internal Medicine
Endocrinology Unit
State University Hospital
De Pintelaan 185
B-9000 Belgium

1
THE HISTORY AND EXAMINATION OF THE INFERTILE MALE

Anne M. Jequier

The evaluation of male infertility does not begin with a semen analysis – it begins with the history and clinical examination of the infertile man. A semen analysis can only occasionally provide the clinician with a diagnosis while a careful history and clinical examination very often reveals the cause of a man's infertility. Diagnosis in infertility is essential for an accurate prognosis and for rational therapy.

However, the history and clinical examination must be relevant to all the different causes of infertility in the male and thus a knowledge of the pathological processes that lead to infertility is very necessary. As with any branch of medicine, the diagnosis of the cause of male infertility is essential for its treatment.

THE HISTORY

Infertility is a problem of a couple, not of an individual (Steinberger and Rodrigues-Rigau, 1983). Thus both partners must be involved in all the facets of the problem. For this reason, the history is taken from an infertile man in the presence of his partner. The history must be taken in quiet, calm surroundings, and there must be no apparent constraints on the clinician's time. Both partners must be allowed, and indeed encouraged, to question the clinician.

The length of infertility must be ascertained, together with any history of previous pregnancies. The outcome of these pregnancies must also be known. The age of the patient, though less important in infertility in the male than in the female, must also be obtained from the history.

It is important to enquire about the general health of an infertile man. A history of chronic chest disease in a man with azoospermia (Young's Syndrome) is almost diagnostic of obstruction. General symptoms, including weight loss may suggest different types of generalised disease. Micturition symptoms may also suggest a variety of different causes of male infertility.

The past history is also very important. Previous episodes of testicular trauma, testicular swelling, orchitis and testicular maldescent may all result in spermatogenic failure. Mumps, a much overstated cause of male infertility, will only cause spermatogenic failure when it occurs in adults and is associated with

1

bilateral orchitis. However, previous operations for hernia, hydrocele, and even testicular maldescent may all cause ductal obstruction (Hanley, 1955). Pelvic and para-aortic surgery may also interfere with both potency and the neurological mechanisms involved in ejaculation (Fossa *et al.*, 1985).

A history of genital tuberculosis and of sexually transmitted disease is also very relevant to male infertility but it is of interest that gonorrhoea now seems to be a relatively uncommon cause of epididymo-orchitis and sterility (Jequier, 1986). Tuberculous epididymitis is now rarely seen in Western Europe.

A history of any present medication is also of relevance. Certain drugs, notably compounds such as salazopyrine (Levi *et al.*, 1979) and even cimetidine (Van Thiel *et al.*, 1979) may impair semen quality while other substances, especially the antihypertensives, may interfere with both potency and ejaculation. Recent surgery or a recent severe medical illness will result in stress and these may also result in temporary infertility.

A sexual history must also be obtained. The frequency of intercourse and any history of impotency must be elicited. Loss of libido, even without impotence, may be a pointer to a large number of endocrine causes of infertility. Pain or discomfort in the lower sacrum or perineum may suggest the presence of ejaculatory duct obstruction. The presence of retrograde ejaculation, or ejaculatory failure may be ascertained by a history of absence of ejaculate, or of ejaculate of low volume (Crich and Jequier, 1978). In men with retrograde ejaculation, a 'cloudy' urine may have been noted post-coitally.

It is also of value to determine the patient's occupation, as this can give clues concerning the ingestion of toxins, exposure to irradiation and also to any factor in a patient's work that may induce stress. It is also of value to enquire about alcohol intake as there is now increasing evidence that alcohol may play an important role in the production of male infertility. There is no evidence that smoking, even when excessive, exerts any affect on fertility.

THE EXAMINATION

It is important to carry out a general examination as well as an examination of the genitalia. The signs of normal androgenisation such as beard growth, body hair distribution and androgen-dependent balding must be sought as loss of these signs may denote Leydig cell failure and the other endocrinopathies that cause androgen deficiency. Gynaecomastia, as seen in Klinefelter's Syndrome, (Paulsen *et al.*, 1968) or in men with Leydig cell tumours may be present. The chest should be auscultated and blood pressure taken. Any chest signs suggesting the presence of bronchiectasis may signal the presence of Young's Syndrome or Immobile Cilia Syndrome (Elliasson *et al.*, 1977).

On examination of the abdomen, it is important to note the presence of scars especially in the groins, which may denote previous hernia operations.

Examination of the genitalia, of course, forms the most important part of the examination. The penis and the external meatus must be inspected. The foreskin should be retracted to exclude phimosis and meatal structure which can result in defective ejaculation. The size of the testes must be ascertained. Their size is usually compared with an orchiometer such as that devised by Prader (Prader, 1966) which provides a testis volume in millimetres (Figure 1.1). It is not sufficient to guess the size of the testes for their exact volume is very important diagnostically. Loss of sensation of the testes can occur in primary lesions of the testes and this sign can be of value diagnostically in some patients.

When an obstructive lesion is present in the epididymis, its upper part becomes distended and is easily palpable. This finding is known as 'Bayle's' sign and denotes the presence of an epididymal obstruction (Bayle, 1952). The presence of a hard epididymis may signify the presence of tuberculous epididymitis.

It is also important to palpate each vas deferens. Congenital absence of

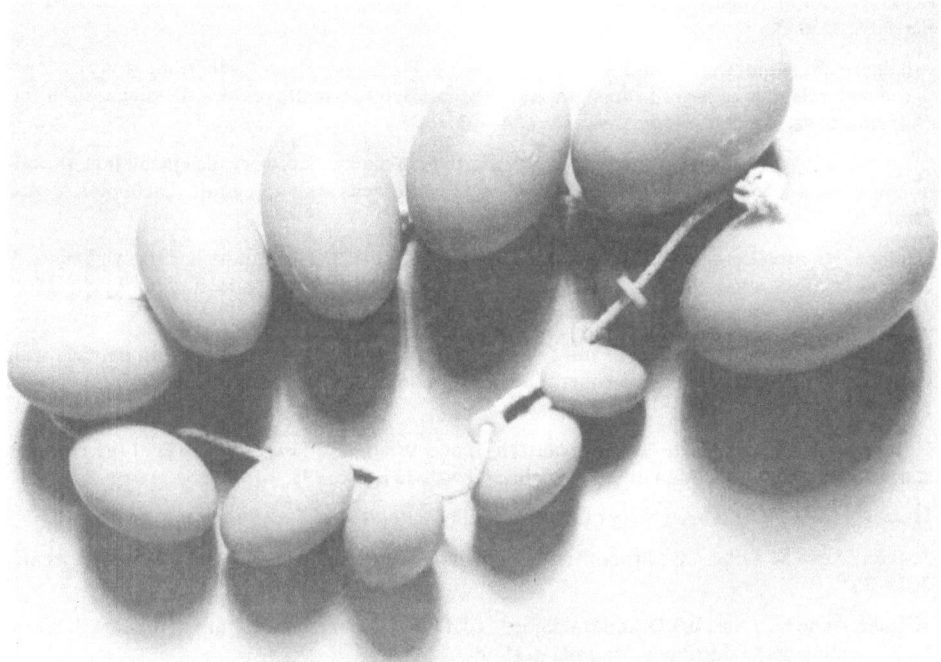

Figure 1.1 A Prader orchiometer, used to determine testicular volume.

the vasa is a well known cause of obstruction of the male genital tract and diagnosing the absence of the vasa will save the patient from unnecessary surgery (Jequier *et al.*, 1985).

Rectal examination only rarely provides any useful information in male infertility. However, if ejaculatory duct obstruction is suspected, it may be possible to palpate the distended seminal vesicles. Occasionally, prostatitis may be a cause of male infertility.

The presence of a varicocoele can only be determined with the patient standing up. The varicocoele, if large, may be palpated directly or during a Valsalva manoeuvre. Characteristic bruit may be elicited by using Doppler apparatus (Greenberg *et al.*, 1977) and even very small varicocoeles can also be demonstrated thermographically.

The history and clinical examination are vital for the correct evaluation of an infertile male. From the history and clinical examination a diagnosis can be made. Investigations can then confirm or refute that diagnosis, and a semen analysis may be used to determine the severity of the lesion. Only when the diagnosis is made, can the correct management of a couple's infertility be planned and carried out.

References

Bayle, H. (1952). Azoospermia of excretory origin – Proceedings of the Society for the Study of Fertility., 4, 30–38

Comhaire, F., Monteyne, R. and Kunnen, M. (1976). The value of scrotal thermography as compared with selective retrograde venography of the internal spermatic vein for the diagnosis of the 'Subclinical' varicocoele. *Fertil. Steril.*, 27, 694–701

Crich, Joan P. and Jequier, Anne M. (1978). Infertility in men with retrograde ejaculation: the action of urine on sperm motility and a simple method for achieving antegrade ejaculation. *Fertil. Steril.*, 30, 572–6

Eliasson, R., Mossberg, B., Camner, and Afzelius, B.A. (1977). The immobile cilia syndrome. A congenital ciliary abnormality as an aetiologic factor in chronic airway infections and male infertility. *N. Engl. J. Med.*, 297, 1

Fossa, S.D., Ous, S., Abyholm, T. and Loeb, M. (1985). Post-treatment fertility in patients with testicular cancer. Influence of retroperitoneal lymph node dissection on ejaculatory potency. *Br. J. Urol.*, 57, 204–09

Greenberg, S.H., Lipshultz, L.I., Morganroth, J. and Wein, A.J. (1977). The use of the Doppler stethoscope in the evaluation of varicocoeles. *J. Urol.*, 117, 196–298

Hanley, H.G. (1955). The surgery of male infertility. *Annals Roy. Coll.Surg. Engl*, 17, 159–183

Jequier, Anne M. (1985). Obstructuive Azoospermia: a study of 102 patients. *Clin. Reprod. Fertil.*, 3, 21–36

Jequier, Anne M,., Ansell, I.D. and Bullimore, N.J. (1985). Congenital absence of the vasa deferentia presenting with infertility. *J. Androl.*, 6, 15–19

Levi, A.J., Fisher, A.M., Hughes, L. and Hendry, W.F. (1979). Male infertility due to sulphasalazine. *Lancet*, 2, 276–8

Paulsen, C.A., Gordon, D.L., Carpenter, R.W., Gandy, H.M. and Drucker, W.D. (1968). Klinefelters syndrome and its variants: a hormonal and chromosomal study. Recent *Progress in Hormone Research*, 24, 321–52

Prader, A. (1966). Testicular size: assessment and clinical importance. *Triangle*, 7, 240–3

Steinberger, E. and Rodrigues–Rigau, L.J. (1983). The infertile couple. *J. Androl.*, 4, 111–18

Van Thiel, D.H., Gavaler, J.S., Smith, W.I and Paul, G. (1979). Hypothalamic–pituitary–gonadal dysfunction in men using cimetidine. *N. Engl. J. Med.*, 300, 1012–15

2
THE HISTORY OF MALE INFERTILITY AND COMPUTER ASSISTED MANAGEMENT OF THE INFERTILE MALE

F.H. Comhaire, F.A. Schoonjans, E. Rombaut, P.J. Rowe and T.T. Farley

INTRODUCTION

A couple is arbitrarily considered infertile when the partners have been unsuccessful in achieving conception after 12 months or more of 'exposure to the risk of pregnancy'. Of 7570 such couples evaluated according to a standard protocol, 65% presented female pathology, 48% male pathology, and in 24% of couples abnormalities were found in both partners (World Health Organization, 1984, 1985). The prevalence of coincidental pathology in both partners was 10-fold higher than expected by chance, suggesting that a combination of factors which reduce the fertility of each partner may result in couple infertility. Hence, evaluation of the infertile couple should always include both partners. In this chapter a summary is given of factors in the history which are relevant to male infertility, and a computer program is described for the registration of data and standardized diagnosis.

FACTORS FROM THE HISTORY WITH POSSIBLE INFLUENCE ON FERTILITY

History of medical disease

Diabetes mellitus and certain **neurological diseases** are known to be associated with ejaculatory disturbances, usually retrograde ejaculation or anejaculation. If ejaculation occurs normally, the prevalence of azoospermia or abnormal semen tends to be higher than in male partners of infertile couples not presenting these diseases, but the differences are not statistically significant. (Table 2.1).

A history of **chronic respiratory tract disease** or **bronchiectasis** is commonly associated with azoospermia due to obstruction of sperm transport, as a result of fibrocystic degeneration of the epididymis or of fibrosis of the vas deferens. Other patients present extreme asthenozoospermia as part of the 'immobile cilia syndrome' or Young's syndrome which are characterized by impair-

5

ment of cilial function of the spermatozoa and of the ciliated cells in the nasal mucosa and epithelium of the upper respiratory tract.

Table 2.1 Factors in the history with possible influence on male fertility

	% of cases with AZOOSPERMIA if factor		% of cases with ABNORMAL SEMEN quality if factor	
	absent	present	absent	present
Diabetes mellitus	7.3	16.7	46.5	60.0
Neurological disease	7.3	12.2	46.5	51.2
Bronchiectasis	7.2	32.0*	46.5	82.4*
High Fever	7.3	5.2	46.4	64.4*
Long term medication	7.2	12.3*	46.4	52.9
Urinary tract infection	7.2	8.9	45.3	60.1*
Sexually transmitted disease				
one episode	7.2	7.6	45.7	50.4*
several episodes	7.2	9.0	45.7	54.4*
Epididymitis	7.1	17.3*	46.1	70.2*
Testicular injury	7.1	12.6*	46.2	56.9*
Testicular torsion	7.3	18.2*	46.5	88.9*
Testicular maldescent				
unilateral	6.8	20.8*	46.1	65.7*
bilateral	6.8	40.8*	46.1	75.9*
Excessive alcohol				
consumption	7.2	9.6	46.4	51.8

* = differences significant at 5% level

High fever (over 38°C) can temporarily suppress sperm production with oligozoospermia, but is not related to azoospermia.

Certain **long-term medical treatments** are known to suppress spermatogenesis, resulting in permanent or temporary azoospermia. Among these, alkylating cytostatic medication and sex hormones such as oestrogens, progestogens, high dose androgens, anabolic steroids and LHRH analogues are to be mentioned. Sulfapyridine is an example of a drug which impairs semen quality by causing abnormal sperm morphology. The effect of other medications suspected to interfere with sperm production, such as nitrofurane derivatives and cimetidine, remains to be proven.

History of surgery

Surgery of the urethral tract including prostatectomy and interventions for hypospadias, for bladder neck sclerosis or for urethral strictures, may interfere with normal ejaculation. Other operations may influence gonadal function or sperm transport, e.g. vasectomy, sympathectomy or repair of inguinal hernia.

History of Infection

A history of **urinary tract infection** with symptoms of dysuria, pyuria, haematuria, urgency or frequency of micturition, is found more commonly in men with abnormal semen quality, but not in patients with azoospermia.

A single episode, but more evidently, recurrent episodes of **sexually transmitted disease** increase the prevalence of abnormal semen quality, particularly abnormal sperm motility and morphology.

A history of **epididymitis**, which is often associated with chronic male accessory gland infection, results in a clearly increased incidence of oligozoospermia and azoospermia.

History of accquired damage

Several diseases may cause **testicular damage**. Among these orchitis, due to infectious parotiditis or other causes, testicular torsion, or injury with scrotal haemorrhage or haematuria, have a high prevalence of azoospermia or severe oligozoospermia.

If the patient has undergone **treatment for varicocele**, this should be registered and the effectiveness of treatment should be evaluated by means of scrotal thermography and/or Doppler echography.

History of congenital disease

A history of **testicular maldescent,** as well as the type of treatment and age at which treatment was performed, have major influence on fertility. Patients with such a history have a high prevalence of azoospermia or severe oligozoospermia, particularly if maldescent was bilateral.

History of other factors

The role of certain **environmental factors** requires further study. There is some evidence to suggest that long lasting exposure to high temperature or to certain industrial chemicals, such as carbon disulphide and pesticides, may interfere with spermatogenesis.

The **excessive consumption of alcohol**, as well as the regular **use of drugs** or narcotics may influence semen quality, though effects on spermatogenesis are unpredictable and variable between individuals.

History of sexual function

For the purpose of fertility evaluation, questions concerning **sexual and ejaculatory function** may be restricted to whether the quality of erection is sufficient for intravaginal intercourse, whether coitus takes place with adequate frequency and correct timing, and whether intravaginal ejaculation occurs.

DATA MANAGEMENT AND COMPUTERIZED DIAGNOSIS

The history taking should be completed by general physical examination and

MALE PARTNER

Date of history taking | Day | Month | Year   Date of birth | Day | Month | year

HISTORY OF (IN)FERTILITY

Infertility — ☐ primary / ☐ secondary

Months since last fertilization
Duration of infertility
Previous investigation(s) and/or treatment(s) for infertility — ☐ no | ☐ yes

PATHOLOGY OF TREATMENT(S) WITH POSSIBLE INFLUENCE ON FERTILITY

History of medical disease — ☐ no | ☐ diabetes ☐ chronic respiratory tract disease ☐ neurologic disease | ☐ tuberculosis ☐ fibrocystic disease of the pancreas ☐ other*

History of medical treatment — ☐ no | ☐ yes*
High fever in past 6 months — ☐ no | ☐ yes*
History of surgery — ☐ no | ☐ urethral strictures ☐ prostatectomy ☐ vasectomy ☐ inguinal hernia ☐ sympathectomy | ☐ hypospadias ☐ bladder neck operation ☐ hydrocelectomy ☐ other*

History of urinary infection — ☐ no | ☐ yes*
History of sexually transmitted disease — ☐ no | ☐ syphilis ☐ chlamydia | ☐ gonorrhoea ☐ other*

side: left-right

History of epididymitis — ☐ no | ☐ yes* ☐ ☐
History of pathology possibly causing testicular damage — ☐ no | ☐ orchitis: mumps ☐ ☐ / ☐ orchitis: other* ☐ ☐ / ☐ injury* ☐ ☐ / ☐ torsion* ☐ ☐

History of varicocele treatment — ☐ no | ☐ yes* ☐ ☐
History of testicular maldescent — ☐ no | ☐ yes ☐ ☐
Treatment for testicular maldescent — ☐ none | ☐ medical / ☐ surgical | age at treatment

OTHER FACTORS WITH POSSIBLE INFLUENCE ON FERTILITY

Environmental and/or occupational factors — ☐ no | ☐ heat ☐ toxic factors | ☐ other*
Excess consumption of alcohol — ☐ no | ☐ yes*
Drug abuse — ☐ no | ☐ yes*

SEXUAL AND EJACULATORY FUNCTION

Average frequency of vaginal intercourse per month — ☐ normal | ☐ inadequate
Erection — ☐ normal | ☐ inadequate*
Ejaculation — ☐ normal | ☐ inadequate*

Figure 2.1

GENERAL PHYSICAL EXAMINATION

Height (cm)
Weight (kg)
Blood pressure (mm Hg)

General physical examination	☐ normal	☐ abnormal*
Signs of virilisation	☐ normal	☐ hypoandrogenism*
Gynecomastia	☐ absent	☐ Tanner stage

URO-GENITAL EXAMINATION

| Penis | ☐ normal | ☐ scars | ☐ hypospadias |
| | | ☐ plaques | ☐ other* |

side: left - right

| Testes | ☐ both palpable | non-palpable | ☐ | ☐ |
| Site | ☐ both normal | abnormal* | ☐ | ☐ |

Volume (ml)   ☐☐   ☐☐
                left   right

Epididymes	☐ both normal	thickened	☐	☐
		tender	☐	☐
		cystic	☐	☐
		non-palpable	☐	☐
Vasa deferentia	☐ both normal	thickened	☐	☐
		non-palpable	☐	☐
Scrotal swelling	☐ none	hydrocele	☐	☐
		hernia	☐	☐
Varicocele	☐ none	grade III	☐	☐
		grade II	☐	☐
		grade I	☐	☐
		subclinical	☐	☐
Inguinal examination	☐ normal	lymphadenopathy	☐	☐
		infectious scars	☐	☐
		surgical scars	☐	☐
		hernia	☐	☐
Rectal examination	☐ normal			
- prostate		☐ soft swelling	☐ tender	
		☐ hard swelling	☐ other	
- seminal vesicles		☐ palpable		
Contact thermography	☐ normal	☐ abnormal*		

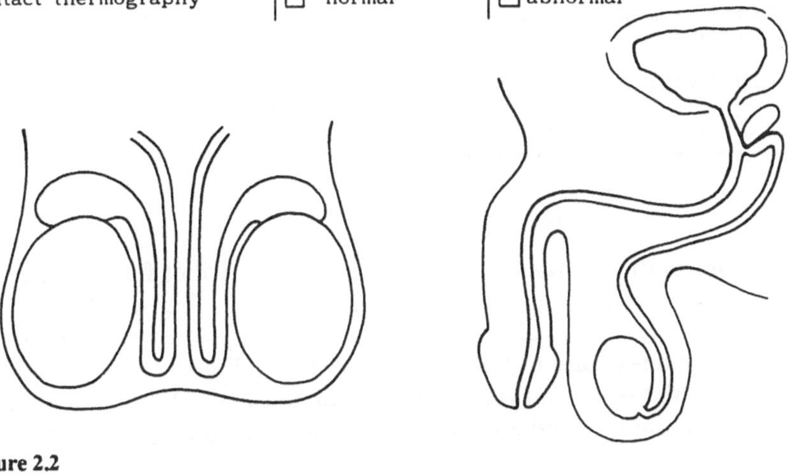

Figure 2.2

careful as well as systematic evaluation of the genital region. These data, together with the results of semen analysis, additional investigations of blood and urine, endocrine analysis, scrotal thermography and/or Doppler echography, elective imaging of the sella turcica, and testicular biopsy are registered in a microcomputer program. The Thoroughbred Operating System serves as carrier for the program which can be run on any IBM compatible microcomputer with a 10 megabyte memory capacity (hard disk).

Entry of the data can be performed by the clinician, by the laboratory, and/or by the secretariat using separate terminals. The data of the patient are either collected on forms (Figures 2.1 and 2.2) or entered directly into the computer. The lay-out of the forms and computer screens are identical and involves both the male and the female partner.

Either the couple number, or the record number, or the name of the male or female partner can be used for identification. The program is extremely user-friendly and does not require any experience since all interactions are given through four function keys and the numeric keys.

For the sake of simplicity every normal response is registered by touching key '1' or the 'ENTER' (carriage return) key; the abnormal response is recorded by touching key '2'. If the clinician wants to return to a previous item

```
SEMEN ANALYSIS (FIRST ANALYSIS)

86001-L    JONES

1. DATE                         : 24/09/87        LAB NUMBER    : 87 1452
   NUMBER OF DAYS SINCE LAST EJACULATION                        : 3 days
ANALYSIS OF SPERMATOZOA                  SEMINAL FLUID ANALYSIS
-----------------------                  ----------------------

 2. CONCENTRATION x 10 6/ml  :  12.7     11. VOLUME (ml)                      :  2.3
 3. MOTILITY - RAPID LINEAR  :  32 %     12. APPEARANCE AND CONSISTENCY  : NORM
 4.          - SLOW LINEAR   :  14 %     13. pH                               :  7.3
 5. NON PROGRESSIVE MOT.     :  21 %     14. BIOCHEMISTRY                     : NORM
 6. IMMOTILE                 :  33 %     15. WHITE BLOOD CELLS x 10 6/ml :  0.2
 7. VIABILITY - % live       :  84 %     16. OTHER ROUND CELLS x 10 6/ml :  0.1
 8. MORPHOLOGY % ideal forms :  26 %     17. CULTURE                     : NEG
 9. MAR/IB-test % positive   :   0 %     18. ADDITIONAL ANALYSIS         : YES
10. AGGLUTINATION            : NONE

SEMEN CLASSIFICATION : OLIGOZOOSPERMIA

'CR' TO CONTINUE, IF INCORRECT ENTER LINENUMBER :  ..        F2 = HELP
```

Figure 2.3

in order to control the input and possibly change it, he strikes function-key 'F4'. If he wants to receive explanation concerning any item, the help function-key 'F2' is touched for relevant definitions, technical descriptions or program information. If optional tests are not done, function-key 'F3' is depressed, and if the result of a particular test is not yet available, function-key 'F1' is touched. Inconsistency between data is immediately detected and brought to the attention of the operator.

The results of semen analyses are registered on one single screen (Figure 2.3) which can be completed either via a terminal in the laboratory, or by the clinician. Numeric data or qualitative information are entered for every characteristic of the spermatozoa and of the seminal plasma. The computer evaluates the results in comparison with normal limits stored in a memory file. As soon as results are completed, the semen analysis is classified into one out of eight possible categories. When two semen samples are analysed, the computer selects

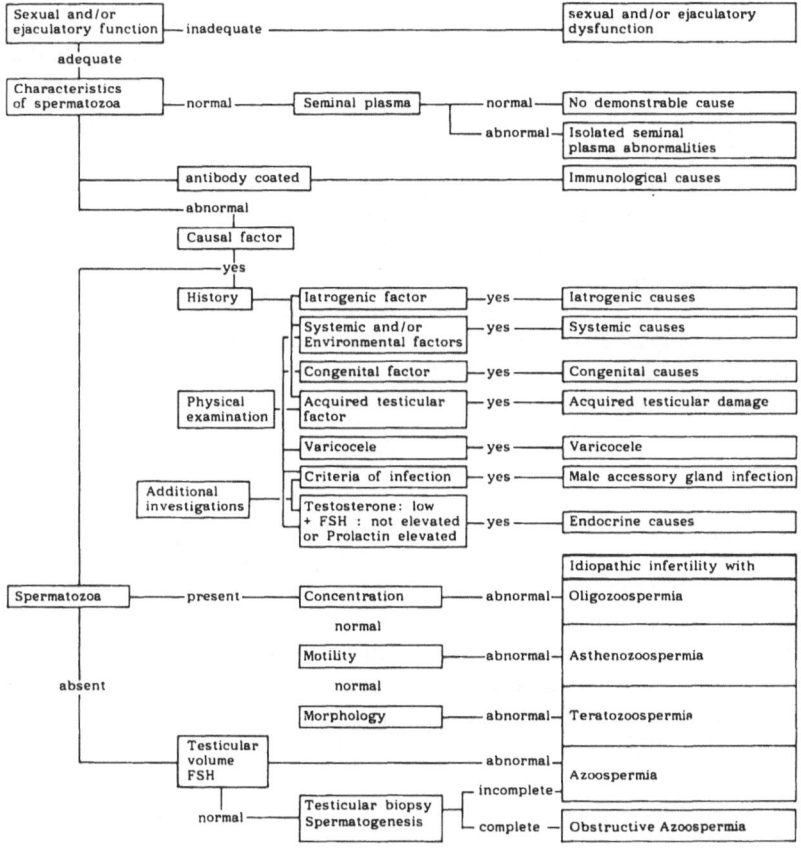

Figure 2.4

the highest ranking of the two which is then used for diagnostic classification.

The clinician is invited to select his diagnosis, which he can compare to standard diagnosis or diagnoses selected by the computer on the basis of a flow chart (Figure 2.4). Moreover, a particular sub-diagnosis is highlighted whenever a more general diagnosis would have been chosen. By entering the number of a diagnosis, the clinician receives information on why that particular diagnosis has been accepted or rejected.

As soon as the results of both the male and the female partner have been recorded, a couple summary appears which lists the diagnosis of both partners and calculates the expected treatment independent pregnancy rate.

Pilot testing of the program in over 400 couples by three centres reveals that the time needed to enter the data is between 5 and 10 minutes for each partner.

A printed report is immediately available, implying additional gain of time and money since there is no more need for secretarial assistance nor file keeping. The clinician can request a printout of each separate screen or a structured summary of data including all numeric and relevant findings as well as the diagnoses.

Storage of data allows the clinician to perform thorough statistical analysis of his entire patient material or of specific subgroups of patients presenting whatever association of characteristics he wishes to study.

Hence, the program serves several purposes, namely data collection and analysis, administration and artificial intelligence. It is a tool for daily clinical work and for teaching.

Further developments of the program include registration of data from the follow-up, programs suggesting patient treatment possibilities, sperm bank administration and donor selection, and a method for the objective measurement of sperm velocity characteristics.

CONCLUSION

History taking gives the key to aetiological diagnosis in approximately one out of eight men with abnormal semen, and in one out of four men in whom a cause for infertility can be detected. History taking should be performed systematically and the registration of data, together with the complete information on further investigations can be done rapidly and conveniently with the help of an extremely user-friendly program for microcomputers. Standardized investigation and diagnosis should improve the quality of management and the success of treatment of male infertility.

ACKNOWLEDGEMENTS

This study was supported by a grant of the World Health Organization, Special Programme of Research, Development and Research Training in Reproduction.

References

World Health Organization. (1984). Workshop on the standardized investigation of the infertile couple. Moderator P. Rowe, co-ordinator M. Darling. In Harrison, R.F., Bonnar, J. and Thompson, W. (eds.) *Fertility and Sterility* p. 427 (Lancaster: MTP Press)

World Health Organization. (1985). 14th Annual Report, p. 119

DISCUSSION

Question: Have you any data on the effects of stress on male fertility?

Comhaire: No.

Question: Did men admitting alcohol abuse have a history of sexual dysfunction?

Comhaire: Generally not. The influence of excessive alcohol consumption on spermatogenesis and testicular hormone production needs further study. The prevalence of both azoospermia and abnormal semen classification was higher in men admitting regular consumption of 60 grammes or more of alcohol per day; the difference with controls was, however, not significant. In men with excessive alcohol consumption the mean serum testosterone concentration was significantly lower if azoospermia or abnormal semen were found, than if the semen was normal. Such a trend was not seen in men without alcohol consumption. This sustains the hypothesis that possible deleterious influence of excessive alcohol consumption on spermatogenesis runs parallel with, or is related to, that on hormone production.

Question: Does post pubertal mumps orchitis have to be bilateral to affect semen quality?

Comhaire: There is some difference between unilateral or bilateral orchitis, as far as effects on spermatogenesis are concerned but both situations cause significant impairment. However, this information is based on history taking and does not include histological examination.

Question: Have you examined men who are very fertile i.e. examining factors that are keeping them fertile?

Comhaire: No. If you were to examine such specific population, other criteria for 'fertility' may be found. We do have data on very fertile donors. These are characterized by the high ATP contents of their semen.

13

3
SEMEN ANALYSIS

T.D. Glover

Unless a man is a semen donor in a donor insemination programme, there is currently no unimpeachable method of predicting his fertility. In biological terms, the production of a baby, following sexual intercourse or donor insemination is not a measure of male fertility, since men with poor semen quality frequently find that they have fathered a child, but could hardly be considered as highly fertile. It is arguable also, that penetration of hamster eggs by human spermatozoa strictly demonstrates their ability to penetrate eggs of that species only and, in any case, gives no indication of zygotic development. Even penetration of human eggs simply represents a step in the reproductive process and early development of a zygote is only a single stage in that process. Fully controlled fertility trials, in the truly experimental sense, obviously cannot be undertaken in man and consequently, an alternative means of assessing human male fertility is required.

A simple method of assessment would be most welcome (how convenient it would be if a single blood sample, for instance, could yield some magical answer), but most clinicians would still question its value without there being some concurrent panacea for treatment. However, uncomplicated answers and facile remedies are at this stage unrealistic because the biology of sperm production and function is multidimensional; not only in terms of physiological parameters but also in terms of the underlying social and evolutionary factors that are involved.

Since semen is the fertilizing substance, it is a logical target for attention in attempts to predict a man's chances of fathering a child (which is what most male patients ask for). This will probably only be possible after a suitable means of assessing human male fertility itself has been devised. So far it has not, so answers to predictive questions, such as 'what are the chances of enough spermatozoa reaching the site of fertilization and of a conception occurring if they do?', must at this time be partly speculative.

Thus, it is reasonable to ask if the analysis of semen serves any useful purpose at all. An answer lies in the fact that even if it has limitations for the accurate prediction of male fertility, it can be used to detect major deficiencies in the male reproductive system. This must surely be of some advantage, because a patient can at least be informed that his semen is significantly deficient, even if suitable treatment may not be immediately at hand. Moreover, if the origin of any defect can be deduced, a rational basis for treatment is more likely to be apparent. Even so, although gross abnormalities such as azoospermia, severe oligozoospermia, serious teratozoospermia, necrozoospermia or asthenospermia are easily recognized, finer interpretation of a semen picture is more difficult. Unobtrusive deficiencies in spermatozoa might easily be missed and the patient's case erroneously categorized as one of 'unexplained infertility'. If, in such cases, in vitro fertilization (IVF) or the application of the gamete intra-fallopian transfer (GIFT) technique also fail, the andrologist is no nearer to knowing what was wrong with the spermatozoa in the first place. The need for very careful semen analysis is thus evident.

Doubtless, there are functional aberrations in spermatozoa that cannot be recognized by contemporary methods of semen analysis, but the purpose of this chapter is to provide some indication of how optimum results might be obtained from some of the semen tests that are presently available. Tests on the spermatozoa themselves will be emphasized, not to diminish the importance of examining seminal plasma, but rather because of the limitations of space and my understanding that the characteristics of seminal plasma will be discussed by other contributors to this book. This also applies to sperm agglutination and other immunological factors.

Typically, after ejaculate volume has been measured, the spermatozoa in a semen sample are examined by estimating total sperm concentration (sperm count); perhaps total sperm number; sperm motility and the incidence of morphological abnormalities. The tests are well known and widely used, but the relative importance of each test is a matter which appears to have received too little attention. The significance of any semen test as an aid to locating the source of a functional defect is important, because it would be fatuous to use it if it proved to be a purely routine or traditional test and to have little diagnostic value.

POSSIBLE SOURCES OF DEFICIENT SPERM PRODUCTION

Testicular abnormalities

The dual function of the testis in producing spermatozoa and serving as an endocrine gland results in it being dependent upon pituitary function. A simplified illustration of the presiding role of the hypophysis, chiefly through its gonadotropins, and the related importance of the hypothalamus, is given in Figure 3.1. The diagram shows that a hypothalamic lesion that is quite remote from the testis (Martini, 1970) (or aberrant signals from other parts of the brain (Scharfetter, 1982)) may jeopardize normal function in the gonad. Abnormality in testosterone feedback (Naftolin et al., 1972; Santen, 1975; Winters et al., 1979a, 1979b) and other disturbances of the synthesis or release of gonadotropins (Johnsen, 1970; Meites, 1970; Glezerman and Lunenfeld, 1982; De Kretser et al., 1983) could all result in abnormal spermatogenesis, whether they concern follicle stimulating hormone (FSH) or luteinizing hormone (LH) production or release. This is well demonstrated in some patients with pituitary tumours and in changes that accompany old age (Baker and Hudson, 1983).

Inside the testis, the absence of protein hormone receptors, or the numerical reduction, desensitization or down regulation of such receptors (Catt and Dufau, 1978; Smals *et al.*, 1983) would also interfere with the normal production of spermatozoa, as would the absence or desensitization of androgen recep-

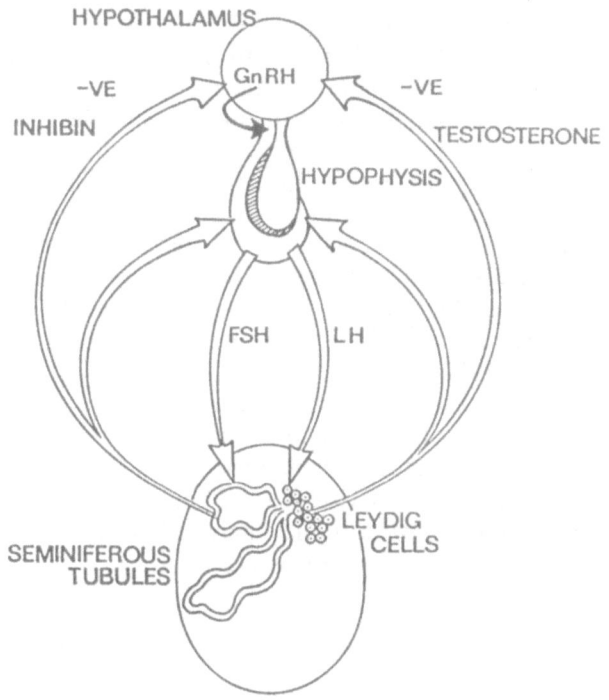

Figure 3.1   Diagrammatic representation of the hypothalamo-hypophysial-testicular axis demonstrating the self-limiting control of the hypophysis over the testis and thus indicating that abnormal testicular function may have its origin at a site quite remote from the gonad, e.g. the hypothalamus or the pituitary [see text]. Gonadotrophin releasing hormone (GnRH); Follicle stimulating hormone (FSH); Luteinizing (interstitial cell stimulating) hormone (LH).

tors (Bardin *et al.*, 1975) in the seminiferous tubules (Steinberger, 1971).

In addition, the interchange of activity between the tubular and intertubular compartments of the testis (Risbridger *et al.*, 1981) and intercellular communication in the seminiferous tubules (Eusebi *et al.*, 1983) could be disrupted, Sertoli cell function (Ritzèn *et al.* 1981; Rich and De Kretser, 1983) could be impaired or, within the germinal epithelium itself, disturbances could occur at the level of spermatogonial multiplication, during the different phases of meiosis (especially meiotic prophase), or during maturation of the spermatid.

There are, therefore, many different sites in the whole hypothalamo-hypophyseal-gonadal axis at which abnormality could give rise to azoospermia, oligozoospermia, or functional abnormalities in spermatozoa. Furthermore, complex cell divisions within the germinal epithelium render the process of spermatogenesis exceptionally vulnerable to error (Cohen, personal communication) and consequent loss or abnormality of spermatozoa.

Abnormalies of spermatozoa occurring within the male tract

The above abnormalities, whatever their main cause, are ultimately testicular in origin (primary abnormalities). Damage to spermatozoa may also occur, however, during their maturation in the epididymis, possibly during transit to the pelvic urethra in seminal emission, and in the ultimate mixing with seminal plasma during ejaculation. These abnormalities may be labelled as 'secondary' abnormalities. On the face of it, the recognition of an abnormality as being primary or secondary might seem important, but in making predictions it is only true if a difference in functional significance between the two can be proven. Such functional differences have not been demonstrated in human spermatozoa, although correlations between specific sperm characteristics and fertility have long been recognized in animals, such as bulls, that are specially selected for reproductive purposes (Bishop et al., 1954).

Characteristics of the ejaculates of successful semen donors should be a useful guide as to what may be regarded as 'good quality' in a human semen sample. But the difficulty encountered here is variability in quantitative estimates produced by different laboratories. Collection of data, therefore, should ideally be made by computer unless two or more analysts have had an opportunity to synchronize their techniques in terms of reproducibility.

Treatment of the infertile male

Most andrologists will acknowledge that attempts to treat the infertile human male are generally frustrating. Opinions differ about the validity of varicocoelectomy (Fenster and McLoughlin, 1982; Aafjes and Van der Vijver, 1985; Ayodeji and Baker, 1986; Vermeulen et al., 1986). Scrotal cooling is contentious (and probably valueless) and hormone therapy is capricious. FSH treatment for azoospermic patients, provided circulating plasma levels of the hormone are not elevated, may have some merit, but there is no serious physiologically based rationale for the use of steroids in male infertility and gonadotrophins and nonsteroidal agents such as clomiphene appear to yield variable results. If clomiphene does prove to be beneficial, it is usually only transitorily so and may well result, in oligozoospermia for example, in producing more defective spermatozoa than were present in the first place. If the spermatozoa of an oligospermic patient are physiologically deficient, it seems counter-productive to create more of them by means of systemic treatment.

This applies even more to treatment with gonadotrophin releasing hormone (GnRH). Here, since pulsatile delivery currently appears to be the only effective form of administration (Hoffman and Crowley, 1983; Keogh et al., 1984) and is, therefore, expensive and burdensome to the patient, only a fairly certain outcome would justify its regular use.

This dismal record may be the result of many reproductive disorders being of genetic origin. When they are, some brief improvement might be expected from symptomatic treatment, but the basic cause will be obscured and not addressed. For example, an oligozoospermic man might luckily father children and the abnormal condition might pass unrecognized until two or even three generations later, when perhaps a son or grandson is referred to an infertility clinic. There would be no means of knowing whether the condition of the son or grandson was congenital or not. Several chromosomal abnormalities might exist that are infinitely less obvious than Klinefelter's syndrome, for instance.

As with other inherited diseases, therefore, a clinician might only hope to contain or control a genetically based male reproductive disorder for a brief period, because an attack on the root cause will at present be beyond his capacity, especially if he is unable to recognize it. Moreover, the wisdom of treating a heritable reproductive disorder might in any case be regarded as questionable.

Such questions are not the province of the seminologist, however, whose primary role is to interpret the picture that a seminal specimen presents. Nevertheless, it would be helpful if specific genetically based disorders could ultimately be identified by means of semen analysis.

THE INTERPRETATION OF SEMEN QUALITY

Rapid assessments of semen quality are usually based upon the subjective estimate of sperm concentration and the vigour with which the spermatozoa appear to be swimming. But is this enough for a worthwhile determination of the quality of an ejaculate, even if a diagnosis of abnormality rather than a prediction of fertility is being sought? Evidence suggests that even from a cursory glance, extremes of quality in semen, that is, either 'excellent' or 'very poor', may quickly and easily be recognized. But the majority of semen samples referred for analysis fall somewhere between these two extremes, so that some definition of 'acceptable quality' is needed. This demands an appropriate range of values for the different semen tests. Data on the lowest quality of semen produced in a large population of successful semen donors could be used to set a lower limit of acceptability. The colligation of such data is probably necessary because there is always some quantitatively recognizable deficiency in a human semen sample. The level at which an andrologist should try to determine the source of an abnormality in semen is, therefore, the point at issue. Sperm concentration demonstrates the problem clearly, since patients with 5 million spermatozoa/ml or even less have been known to father children. So what is the lowest sperm count that can be accepted before an andrologist should be suspicious of something being seriously wrong and endeavour to locate the source of the problem? Should this be when the count is down to 50 million/ml or 20 million/ml?

These are difficult questions to answer, especially when sperm count and a subjective assessment of motility are frequently the only two criteria in a report on semen quality that receive serious attention. Other characteristics of the semen may give some clue. The next question that arises might then be whether or not any particular semen test is more meaningful than another. There is evidence that sperm motility, if properly estimated, is important (Overstreet and Katz, 1977) and good semen donors almost always have a good sperm count combined with a high proportion of spermatozoa swimming in a straight line and showing minimum lateral displacement of the sperm head which normally rolls round its longitudinal axis (Phillips, 1982). (Since there are a number of different swimming patterns displayed by spermatozoa in a semen sample, this type of motility will be referred to here, for simplicity, as Type 1 motility). It is therefore, important to recognize that not all spermatozoa showing progressive motility are swimming in a straight line.

Table 3.1 Relationship between the incidence of spermatozoa showing Type 1 motility (see text) and the results of post coital tests, when hostile mucus did not appear to be involved

Quality of post coital test	Number of tests	Total% motile spermatozoa ($\pm$ SE)	% spermatozoa showing Type 1 motility (See text)
Good (+/+)	28	53 ± 4	32 ± 4
Poor (+/-)	22	44 ± 4*	17 ± 4**

*No significant difference
**Significant difference (p < 0.01)
Statistical tests used here were the Student's t-test and the Wilcoxon-Mann-Whitney rank sums test.

Table 3.2 Relationship of different parameters of sperm motility, showing sperm speed and flagellar beat, are positively correlated and amplitude of beat is negatively correlated with them

Type of motility	Number of spermatozoa examined	Speed (μm/s $\pm$ SE)	Frequency of flagellar beats/s ($\pm$ SE)	Amplitude of flagellar beats (μm $\pm$ SE)
Type 1 (see text)	20	35.75 ± 2.6	10.95 ± 0.8	4.45 ± 0.3
Head waving	21	32.10 ± 2.5	8.10 ± 0.6	5.20 ± 0.3
Yawing (of the head	8	20.95 ± 2.1	5.00 ± 1.0	5.40 ± 0.5
Whiplash (darting) movement	9	17.00 ± 2.0	3.90 ± 0.6	6.00 ± 0.3

Calculated correlations have shown that speed and flagellar frequency correlate positively [$r = 0.68$($p < 0.001$)], track width and amplitude of beat also [$r = 0.39$($p < 0.001$)], whilst amplitude of flagellar beat and frequency of beat are inversely related [$r = -0.41$($p < 0.001$)], and track width and frequency of beat are also negatively correlated [$r = -0.49$ ($p < 0.001$)].

The standard of post-coital tests seems to be more closely related to the incidence of spermatozoa showing Type 1 motility than to the total percentage of progressively motile spermatozoa (that is, when hostile mucus is not involved).

There is also evidence that spermatozoa showing Type 1 motility are hydrodynamically the most efficient type (Burgess and Glover, 1987).

If Type 1 motility reflects the integrity of flagellar function, a method of measuring it would be helpful. This kind of spermatozoon swims in a straight line

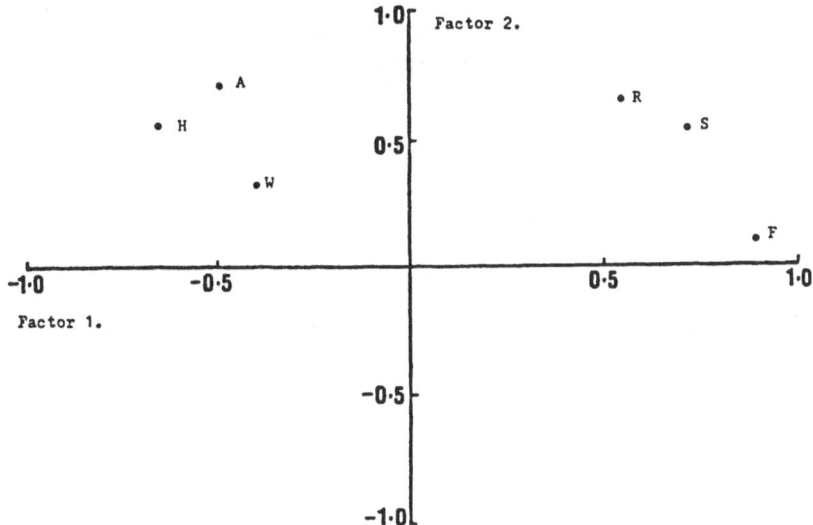

Figure 3.2 Factor matrix resulting from applying Factor Analysis to six factors that contribute to forward propulsion in a spermatozoon. The technique uses a principal factor without iterations (repeated calculations) [Burgess and Glover, 1987]. Amplitude of flagellar beat (A); Head amplitude (H); Wavelength (W); Rate of (head) rotation (R); Speed (S); Wave frequency (F).

and shows minimal displacement of the sperm head. However, there are different degrees of head displacement even in straight swimming spermatozoa, so that qualitative recognition of Type 1 motility in a semen sample is not easy.

A number of factors combine to propel a spermatozoon forward in the most efficient way possible, which means that there are a number of different dimensions of sperm movement also. Some of these are positively correlated, but correlates such as rate of head rotation and sperm speed, head amplitude (lateral displacement of the sperm head), wave amplitude, wavelength and frequence of flagellar beat, may only represent a fraction of the total number of dimensions involved.However, another statistical method, known as Factor Analysis (a principal components analysis technique), can be used to determine relationships between all the variables, since it is a multidimensional analytical system (Du Toit *et al.*, 1980). When applied to sperm motility, the analysis demonstrates that many of the relevant variables are associated with wave frequency (Burgess and Glover, 1982). But of particular importance, is the fact that six major parameters of sperm movement (wave amplitude, head amplitude, wavelength, sperm speed, rate of rotation and wave frequency) fall into two distinct groups of three along a single factor (Factor 1) (Figure 3.2). This means that it is unnecessary to measure all of these factors, in order to obtain a meaningful assessment of motility in a spermatozoon. Only two of them really need to be chosen and since sperm speed and head amplitude are widely separated along Factor 1, they would seem to be the two parameters of choice in this regard.

Obviously, quantitative assessments of this kind are not usually made in the average laboratory, which further suggests that some of the most useful criteria of sperm function may escape attention when routine methods of semen analysis are used.

However, Figure 3.3 shows that different methods of assessing motility, including the incidence of progressively motile spermatozoa, the percentage of

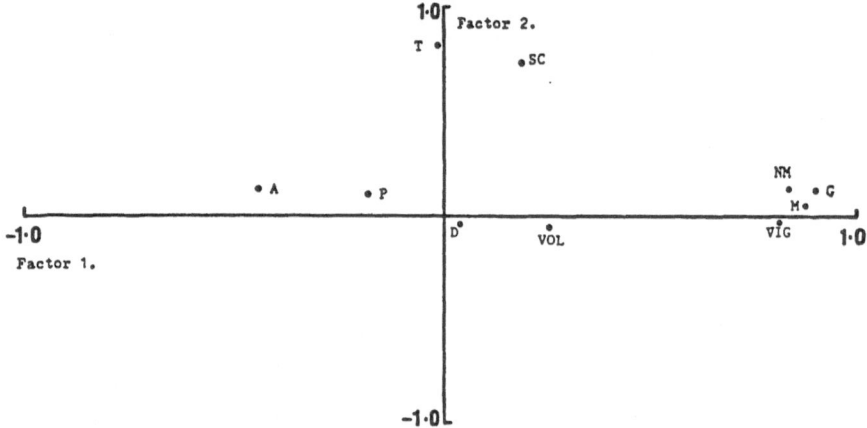

Figure 3.3 Factor matrix obtained from applying Factor Analysis to the following criteria for testing semen quality: % morphologically abnormal spermatozoa (A); % dead spermatozoa (D); volume of ejaculation (VOL); sperm count (SC); incidence of pus cells (P); % spermatozoa with Type 1 motility (NM); total % progressively motile spermatozoa (M); grade of motility (G); vigour (subjective assessment) of spermatozoa (VIG). Testis size (T) was included in the analysis just for interest. The wide distribution of the different criteria of semen quality is to be noted [see text].

spermatozoa showing Type 1 motility (quantitative assessments) and 'grade' of motility and vigour (qualitative assessments), are clustered fairly closely together. This means that there is little variation between results obtained by any of these tests, so that they are all likely to yield a similar result. The suggestion here, therefore, is that a qualitative assessment of motility is useful and may be all that is needed.

Sperm motility, however important it might be, is nevertheless, only one dimension of semen quality, and the application of factor analysis to other semen test characteristics yields a different picture (Figure 3.3). If applied to the most conventional tests of sperm quality, other than motility, factor analysis shows a much wider distribution of variables. Indeed, although a direct relationship between testis size and sperm count is evident in Figure 3.3, there is no clear pattern of relationship between other variables (i.e. between the different semen tests). Overall, Figure 3.3 demonstrates an almost random distribution of parameters. Sperm morphology, for example, appears to have no relationship to other parameters and this applies almost as much to semen volume. In isolation, therefore, none of the criteria shown in Figure 3.3 can be relied upon to provide an accurate reflection of semen quality. In turn, this infers that if a balanced interpretation of a semen sample is to be achieved, all the tests used in the analysis should be applied. Hence, the use of one or even two criteria is inadequate and might well prove deceptive, since the results of different semen tests differ so widely in their contribution to variance. But because the value of one test does not correlate well with that of another, it should not be rejected as being useless. Some criteria of semen quality will correlate positively with others, some will be negatively correlated, and yet most will show no significant relationship to each other whatsoever, or, for that matter, with evidence of fertility.

Sperm morphology, for example, has been shown to have little relationship to pregnancy rate (Zaini et al., 1984), but if it is selected alone with no reference to other semen characteristics, the lack of a relationship tells us very little. If a morphological deformity is serious, the relevant spermatozoon is not likely to be functionally normal, so sperm morphology cannot be totally disregarded as a potentially significant semen test.

Morphological defects in spermatozoa are often observed alongside a heavy load of seminal leukocytes. This observation might at once indicate an infection of the reproductive apparatus resulting in the production of abnormal spermatozoa. But, if, as is often the case, the defect is in the sperm heads, this explanation is unconvincing. How far variations in the nature of seminal plasma might influence sperm morphology is also unclear and no sound information is available on the possible effect of 'alien' cells such as leukocytes, or even organisms themselves, upon sperm structure. Certainly pus cells may be seen phagocytozing spermatozoa. Here again, therefore, precise interpretation is not easy.

Table 3.3 Correlations between the percentage of 'live morphologically normal' spermatozoa and other parameters of semen quality

Semen characteristic	Number of patients	Correlation coefficient	Significance
Total % motility	42	0.4128	Significant, $p < 0.01$
Type 1 motility (see text)	63	0.3208	Significant, $p < 0.01$
% Dead spermatozoa	29	0.1100	Not significant
Sperm count ($\times 10^6$/ml)	29	-0.4001	Significant, $p < 0.05$
Semen volume (ml)	59	-0.0737	Not significant

Our own experience is that estimates of the total number of 'live morphologically normal' spermatozoa (estimated from smears stained with aqueous nigrosin and eosin differential stain; (Campbell *et al.*, 1956)) is a more useful criterion of semen quality rather than the total proportion of morphologically abnormal forms.

Estimates of live morphologically normal spermatozoa are not only more reproducible, but show a close relationship to the incidence of spermatozoa showing Type 1 motility, as well as to the total percentage of motile spermatozoa (Table 3.3).

Variations in semen volume should also receive attention in efforts to identify the source of seminal defects. Reduced semen volume may indicate inflammation or fibrosis of the prostate, whilst large volumes may signify an inflammatory condition of the seminal vesicles. Chemical tests may also be applied. Depressed citric acid content (Mann, 1964), for example, may demonstrate failure of prostatic function and a high incidence of leukocytes may confirm the condition. Yet variations in semen volume might also reflect differences in the force of seminal emission (Cross and Glover, 1958) or in the integrity of the ejaculatory reflex (Scharfetter, 1982). Semen volume declines with frequent ejaculation, for instance. The need to look at semen volume alongside other features of the semen is thus underscored. Of particular value is the relationship of semen volume to sperm count and since both are strikingly influenced by ejaculation frequency, a suitable fixed period of sexual abstinence is essential, before a semen sample is examined (WHO Report, 1980).

CONCLUSIONS

An analogy has been drawn between the assessment of a semen sample and an identikit picture (Glover, 1984) and it is also similar to a jigsaw puzzle. In all three cases, it is difficult to comprehend the whole picture from the observation of a single piece.

The data presented in this chapter should leave little doubt that the interpretation of semen quality is complex and that signs provided by the different tests are sophisticated. In spite of extensive research, the study of spermatozoa, their production, ripening and ultimate functional behaviour, is still in its infancy. There is so much that we do not know about spermatozoa and it is fanciful to expect that, at this stage of our knowledge, we might be able to give a precise prediction about what any of them is likely to do in the female tract or which of them can definitely achieve conception and yield a normally developing fetus. Because of this, traditional semen tests may in some ways be regarded as an encumbrance, even though more accuracy and reproducibility will doubtless result from computerization. Better semen tests than we have at present and better interpretation of existing tests are both required, if semen analysis is to become anything more than a casual guide to man's fertility.

As in any scientific investigation, accuracy and consistency of results are vital. Nevertheless, a qualitatively based interpretation of a semen picture might well be more useful to a clinician than a report that gives precise quantitative data, without any attempt at elucidation.

All the indications are, that 'semen appraisal' should be the dominant aim and until more attention is focussed on it, 'semen analysis' will continue to be of more limited value than is often recognized. Much more debate on the question of interpretation of semen pictures, therefore, seems to be warranted, together with fundamental research on the biology of spermatozoa, which might lead to some new and more valuable semen tests being developed.

ACKNOWLEDGEMENTS

Data presented in this chapter have been selected from research supported by the Australian National Health and Medical Research Council. I wish to thank Dr T.R. Burgess for laboratory assistance and for his unfailing willingness at all times to discuss the results we have obtained. I also thank Dr J.F. Hennessey for allowing us access to material through the Queensland Fertility Group in Brisbane for carrying out the post-coital tests referred to in Table 3.1.

References

Aafjes, J.H. and Van der Vijver, J.C.M. (1985). Fertility of men with and without varicocoele. *Fertil. Steril.*, **43**, 901-4

Ayodeji, O. and Baker, H.W.G. (1986). Is there a specific abnormality of sperm morphology in men with varicocoeles? *Fertil. Steril.*, **45**, 839-42

Baker, H.W.G. and Hudson, B. (1983). Changes in the pituitary-testicular axis with age. In De Kretser, D.N., Burger, H.G., and Hudson, B. (eds.) *The Pituitary and the Testis*. (Berlin: Springer Verlag)

Bardin, C.W., Janne, O., Bullock, L.P. and Jacob, S.T. (1975). Physicochemical and biological properties of androgen receptors. In French, F.S., Hansson, V., Ritzen, E.M. and Nayfeh, S.N. (eds.) *Hormonal Regulation of Spermatogenesis*. (New York, London: Plenum Press)

Bishop, M.W.H., Campbell, R.C., Hancock, J.L. and Walton, A. (1954). Semen characteristics and fertility in the bull. *J. Agric. Sci.*, **44**, 227-48

Burgess, T.R. and Glover, T.D. (1982). Sperm motility in human semen appraisal. 11th Nat. Cong. Indonesian Soc. of Andrology, Bali. pp. 75-6

Burgess, T.R. and Glover, T.D. (1987). Relationships between swimming patterns in human spermatozoa and some specific features of sperm movement. (In preparation)

Campbell, R.C., Dott, H.M. and Glover, T.D. (1956). Nigrosin eosin as a stain for differentiating live and dead spermatozoa. *J. Agric. Sci.*, **48**, 1-8

Catt, K.J. and Dufau, M.L. (1978). Gonadotrophin receptors and regulation of interstitial cell function in the tests. In O'Malley, B. and L. Birnbaumer, (eds.) *Receptors and Hormone Action*. Vol. 3. (New York, London: Academic Press).

Cross, B.A. and Glover, T.D. (1958). The hypothalamus and seminal emission. *J. Endocrinol.*, **16**, 385-95

De Kretser, D.M., Burger, H.G. and Bremner, W.J. (1983). Control of FSH and LH secretion. In De Kretser, D.M., Burger, H.G. and Hudson, B. (eds.) The Pituitary and Testis. (Berlin: Springer Verlag)

Du Toit, S.H.C., Van Aarde, R.J. and Steyn, A.G.W. (1980). Sex determination of the feral house cat Felis catus using multivariate statistical analyses. *S. Afr. J. Wildl. Res.,* **10,** 82-7

Eusebi, F., Ziparo, E., Fratamico, G., Russo, M.A. and Stefanini, M. (1983). Intercellular communication in rat seminiferous tubules. *Devel. Biol.,* **100,** 249-55

Fenster, H. and McLoughlin, M. (1982). Varicocele: Its role in male infertility. In Bain, J., Schill, W.-B. and Schwarzstein, L. (eds.) *Treatment of Male Infertility.* (Berlin: Springer Verlag)

Glezerman, M. and Lunenfeld, B. (1982). Treatment of male infertilty. In Bandhauer, K. and Frick, J. (eds.) *Disturbances in Male Infertility.* (Berlin: Springer Verlag)

Glover, T.D. (1984). Seminal Identikits: *Plenary Session,* Proc. Fertil. Soc. Australia, 3, 9

Hoffman, A.R. and Crowley, W.F. Jr. (1983). Chronic low-dose pulsatile gonadotropin-releasing hormone treatment for idiopathic hypogonadotropic hypogonadism in men. In *Recent Advances in Male Reproduction: Molecular Basis and Clinical Implications.* (New York: Raven Press)

Johnsen, S.G. (1970). Testicular-pituitary interrelationship. In Rosemberg, E. and Paulsen, C.A. (eds.) *The Human Testis.* (New York, London: Plenum Press)

Keogh, E.J., Dunn, A.G., Vujcich, J. *et al.* (1984). Pulsatile gonadotrophin releasing hormone (GnRH) therapy for azoospermia. *Proc. Fertil. Soc. Australia,* 3, 11

Mann, T. (1964). *The Biochemistry of Semen and of the Male Reproductive Tract.* (London: Methuen)

Martini, L. (1970). Hypothalamic control of gonadotrophin secretion in the male. In Rosemberg, E. and Paulsen, C.A. (eds.) *The Human Testis.* (New York, London: Plenum Press)

Meites, J. (1970). Modification of synthesis and release of hypothalamic releasing factors induced by exogenous stimuli. In Martini, L. and Meites, J. (eds.) *Neurochemical Aspects of Hypothalamic Function.* (New York: Academic Press)

Naftolin, F. Ryan, K.J. and Petro, Z. (1972). Aromatization of androstenedione by the diencephalon. *J. Clin. Endocrinol. Metab.,* **33,** 368-70

Overstreet, J.W. and Katz, D.F. (1977). Sperm transport and selection in the female genital tract. In Johnson, M. (ed.) *Development in Mammals,* Vol. 2. (New York: North-Holland Publishing Co.)

Phillips, D. (1982). Direction of rolling in mammalian spermatozoa. In André J. (ed.) *The Sperm Cell.* (The Hague: Martinus Nijhoff)

Rich, K.A. and De Kretser, D.M. (1983). Spermatogenesis and the Sertoli cell. In De Kretser, D.M., Burger, H.G. and Hudson, B. (eds.) *The Pituitary and Testis.* (Berlin: Springer Verlag)

Risbridger, G.P., Hodgson, Y.M. and De Kretser, D.M. (1981). Mechanism of action of gonadotrophins on the testis. In Burger, H. and De Kretser, D.M. (eds.) *The Testis.* (New York: Raven Press)

Ritzén, E.M., Hansson, V. and French, F.S. (1981). The Sertoli cell. In Burger, H. and De Kretser, D.M. (eds.) *The Testis.* (New York: Raven Press)

Santen, R.J. (1975). Is aromatization of testosterone to estradiol required for inhibition of LH secretion in men? *J. Clin. Invest.,* **56,** 1555-63

Scharfetter, F. (1982). Neurology of male fertility disorders. In Bandhauer, K. and Frick, J. (eds.) *Disturbances in Male Fertility.* (Berlin: Springer Verlag)

Smals, A.G.H., Kloppenberg, P.W.C. and Benraad, Th.J. (1983). Effects of single and multiple chorionic gonadotropin administration on Leydig cell function in man. In *Recent Advances in Male Reproduction: 1 Molecular Basis and Clinical Implications* (New York: Raven Press)

Steinberger, E. (1971). Hormonal control of mammalian spermatogenesis. *Physiol. Rev.,* **51**, 1-22

Vermeulen, A., Vandeweghe, M. and Deslypere, J.P. (1986). Prognosis of subfertility in men with corrected or uncorrected varicocele. *J. Androl.,* **7**, 147-55

W.H.O. Report (1980). *Laboratory Manual for the Examination of Human Semen and Semen-Cervical Mucus Interaction.* Belsey, M.A., Eliasson, R., Gallegos, A.J., Moghissi, K.S., Paulsen, C.A. and Prasad, M.R.N. (eds.) (Singapore: Press Concern)

Winters, S.J., Janick, J., Loriaux, D.L. and Scherins, R.J. (1979a). Studies on the role of sex steroids in the feedback control of gonadotrophin concentration in men. II. Use of the estrogen antagonist clomiphene citrate. *J. Clin. Endocrinol. Metab.,* **48**, 222-7

Winters, S.J., Scherins, R.J. and Loriaux, D.L. (1979b). Studies on the role of sex steroids in the feedback control of gonadotrophin concentration in men. III. Androgen resistance in primary gonadal failure. *J. Clin. Endocrinol. Metab.,* **48**, 553-8

Zaine, A., Jennings, M.G. and Baker, H.W.G. (1984). Relationship between morphology and motility of sperm and fertility in subfertile men. *Proc. Fertil. Soc.* Australia, 3, 9

DISCUSSION

Question: Have you examined the influence of the spermatogenic precursor cells in semen samples, on fertility?

Glover: No. But an excess of them is a strong indicator of spermatogenic disorder.

Question: There are some reports that the quality and quantity of semen produced by masturbation is inferior to that produced at coitus or using other methods of collection such as silastic capsules. Can you comment?

Glover: The whole subject of seminal emission requires further attention. For example, if you receive a sample with a small volume, it is difficult, to ascertain the cause, it may be a result of prostatic fibrosis, congestion of the seminal vesicles or a deficiency of the emission reflex. It is hard to assess what the variations in volume mean, because they may be physiologic in nature or they may even be genetic. Also, semen volume frequently declines with age.

In animals, there is very strong evidence that sexual excitation yields a 'better emission reflex' and it is probably associated with the effects of circulating adrenalin. This may be the case in humans beings also, so masturbation may not be an ideal technique for the collection of semen for analysis, but there are no better ones.

27

There is another problem, which is, that if another technique of semen collection becomes generally accepted, it may be necessary to redefine the currently accepted limits of 'normality' derived from commonly used semen tests.

Question: What is your regime for the number of ejaculates and the interval between ejaculates for a reliable assessment of the nature of a semen profile?

Glover: Most workers agree that one sample is inadequate. We ourselves do not have a standard regime, but generally obtain a profile from 3 or 4 semen samples, unless the semen is of exceptionally good quality, when two samples will usually suffice.

Question: The upper limit of the proportion of morphologically normal sperm in semen samples is extremely variable, some authors quoting as many as 80-90% normal forms in some semen samples. Can you comment on these high levels? Also, would it be best to use a staining method or phase contrast microscopy using wet film preparation to examine sperm morphology?

Glover: This is a very good point. Smearing the sperms then staining them does not appear to affect the morphology. However, it is extremely useful to examine a wet film preparation using phase contrast. The human being has a staggering degree of sperm pleomorphism and this is usually interpreted as reflecting a high level of morphological abnormality. This assumes, of course, that we know what a morphologically normal human sperm looks like and that is a fairly tricky assumption. But we believe that it is important, nevertheless, to try and estimate the total number of morphologically 'normal' live spermatozoa that are regularly being inseminated by an individual at coitus. I think this estimate is helpful in attempting to predict the chances of the individual fathering a child within a reasonable period of time, say a year. But personally, I have never examined a human semen sample that contained as many as 90% 'normal' forms, not even in the semen of our best donors[a].

Gordon Baker in Melbourne has not been able to find any relationship between the incidence of morphologically abnormal spermatozoa in semen and success in achieving a pregnancy. But we do not find this surprising and the evidence from my paper today should serve to deter people in the future from trying to determine the validity of a semen test for its use in isolation, that is, in the absence of other tests on the sample.

Question: How essential is it to know the details of the various sperm abnormalities, for example, coiled tails, large heads and so on?

Glover: We do not really know. Preliminary data in our laboratory tentatively suggest that there may be relationship between a high incidence of very large sperm heads and miscarriage. It would be interesting to know if there is a paternal factor involved in some histories of repeated miscarriage, but at this stage we can do little more than ask the question. However, as I said in my paper, it is more obvious that some defects will prevent a sperm from entering an egg, whilst others, it might be presumed, will permit penetration of an egg, but result in failure of normal development of the zygote.

Question: If there is no history of genital infection and no evidence of polymorphonuclear leucocytes, is there any necessity for a culture to be performed on the semen sample?

Glover: The simple answer, to my mind, is 'No'. We are by no means convinced of the validity of performing routine cultures on semen samples. I suspect it might be largely a waste of time.

Question: Do semen characteristics of one individual vary from week to week?

Glover: Not normally, although this comment excludes variations in general health. The quality of semen of any one individual is remarkably constant, given a constant period of abstinence before examination. In fact, you can recognise some men by the characteristics in their semen!

Semen of doubtful quality, however, may show marked variation between samples from the same individual. This is why it is necessary to examine a number of specimens in an infertility clinic.

Reference

(a)   Katz, D.F., Overstreet, J.W., Samuels, S.J., Niswander, P.W., Bloom, T.O. and Lewis, E.L. Morphometric analysis of spermatozoa in the assessment of human male fertility. *J. Androl.*, **7**, 203-210

4
ROLE OF UROLOGICAL SURGERY

W.F. Hendry

The outflow passages from the testicle become obstructed at different sites (Figure 4.1) – the exact site being in general related to the underlying cause. As a result, obstruction can be classified according to the site of the blockage, taking into account the different patho-physiological processes involved. This is of practical importance, since supplementary medical treatment may be required in addition to surgery. A classification based upon the findings of exploratory scrototomy in 168 patients with azoospermia and normal serum FSH levels (Hendry *et al.*, 1983) is shown in Table 4.1.

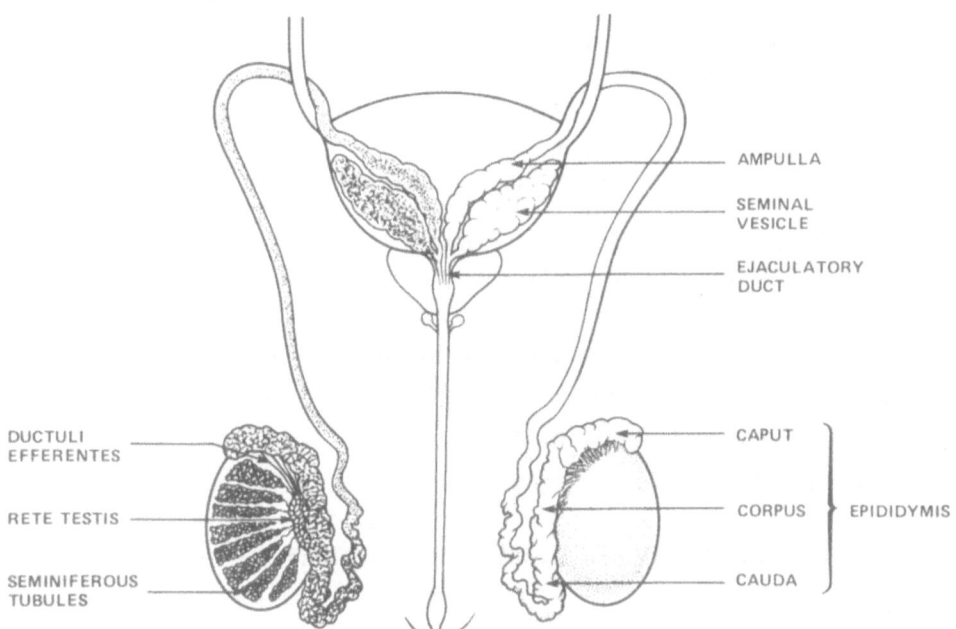

Figure 4.1 The efferent passages of the male genital tract.

31

Table 4.1 Classification of testicular obstruction based on the findings in 167* azoospermic males with normal serum FSH levels (Hendry *et al.*, 1983)

Site of obstruction	Number of cases (%)	Spermato-genesis	Vasogram	Aetiological factors
Empty epididymis	8 (5%)	Absent	Not done	Sertoli cell only
	14 (8%)	Impaired	Not done	Maturation arrest
	2 (1%)	Normal	Not done	Immune orchitis
Caput epididymis	48 (29%)	Normal	Normal	Usually Young's syndrome
Cauda epididymis	34 (20%)	Normal	May be abnormal	Post-infective
Blocked vas	23 (14%)	Normal	Abnormal	Traumatic, infective
Absent vas				
– bilateral	29 (17%)	Normal	Not possible	Congenita
– unilateral	8 (5%)	Normal	Various	Various (Contra-lateral testis)
Ejaculatory duct	1	Normal	Dilated	Congenital, Traumatic

(* The series also included one unclassifiable patient who had had both epididymes excised as treatment for epididymal cysts)

The incidence of each type of obstruction is shown, together with the findings on testicular biopsy and vasography. The commonly related aetiological factors are indicated. In some cases the lesions were asymmetrical, and this is noted when it appears to be a common feature. Although this descriptive classification was worked out in patients with azoospermia, it is equally applicable to unilateral testicular obstruction since its basis is anatomical. The cases are stratified according to:

(i)   the external appearances of the epididymis when examined with magnifying spectacles or operating microscope,

(ii)   the findings on vasography, and

(iii)   the results of testicular biopsy.

CLASSIFICATION OF TESTICULAR OBSTRUCTION

Empty epididymes

In most of these cases, there is absent or impaired spermatogenesis which has not been reflected by elevation of serum FSH levels; occasionally there is gonadotrophin deficiency which may respond to medical therapy. Rarely, there

is normal spermatogenesis associatedwith very high antisperm antibody titres (1024 or greater). Testicular biopsy may show focal mononuclear cell infiltrates indicating that this is a form of auto-immune orchitis, which may respond to prednisolone therapy (see below).

Caput epididymis

This is the largest single group comprising 29% of all cases. In three-quarters of these patients there is co-existing sinusitis, bronchitis or bronchiectasis an association first noted by Young (1970). The distension of the epididymal tubules is confined to the heads of the epididymis (Figure 4.2), and light microscopy

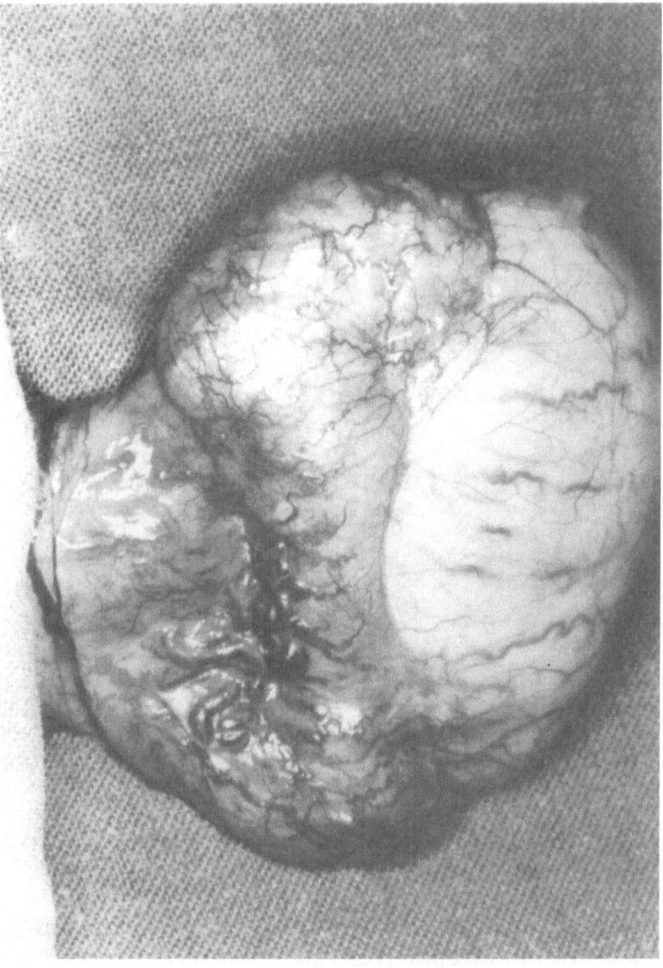

Figure 4.2 Epididymis of a patient with Young's syndrome: note that the tubules are only distended in the caput epididymis, and the rest of the epididymis is empty.

shows that this coincides with the ductuli efferentes, where the epithelium is ciliated; the tubules are filled with inspissated masses of spermatozoa and lipid. Electron microscopy shows that the cilia have the normal 9 + 2 arrangement of microtubules and dynein arms are present (Hendry *et al.*, 1987). Lung mucociliary clearance is impaired (Pavia *et al.*, 1981) even though ciliary beat frequency measured by the technique of Rutland and Cole (1980) is normal. Despite intensive further studies, the aetiology of Young's syndrome remains obscure (Handelsman *et al.*, 1983; Neville *et al.*, 1983). The results of epididymo-vasostomy are generally poor (see below).

Cauda epididymis

This is the appearance commonly seen following infection, which may be gonococcal or chlamydial, due to urinary infection or smallpox, or associated with

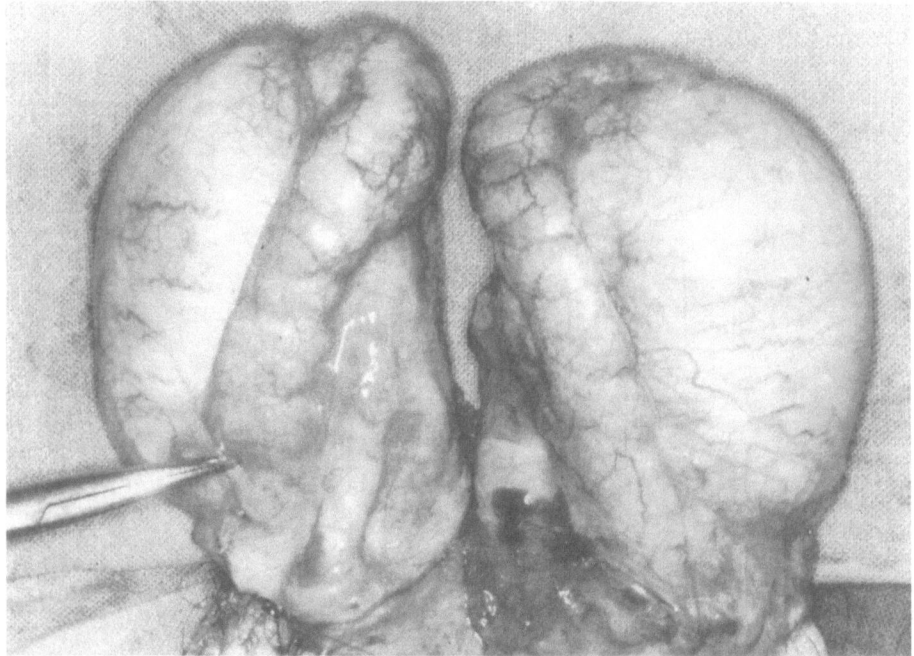

Figure 4.3 Typical appearances of bilateral post-infective caudal blocks, with tubules full throughout the whole length of the epididymes.

a variety of esoteric conditions such as Sandfly fever or Bornholm disease. Typically, the tubules within the epididymis are uniformly distended down to its tail (Figure 4.3). Of course, a similar appearance is seen when the vas is blocked, causing back pressure on the epididymis, and a vasogram is mandatory to ensure

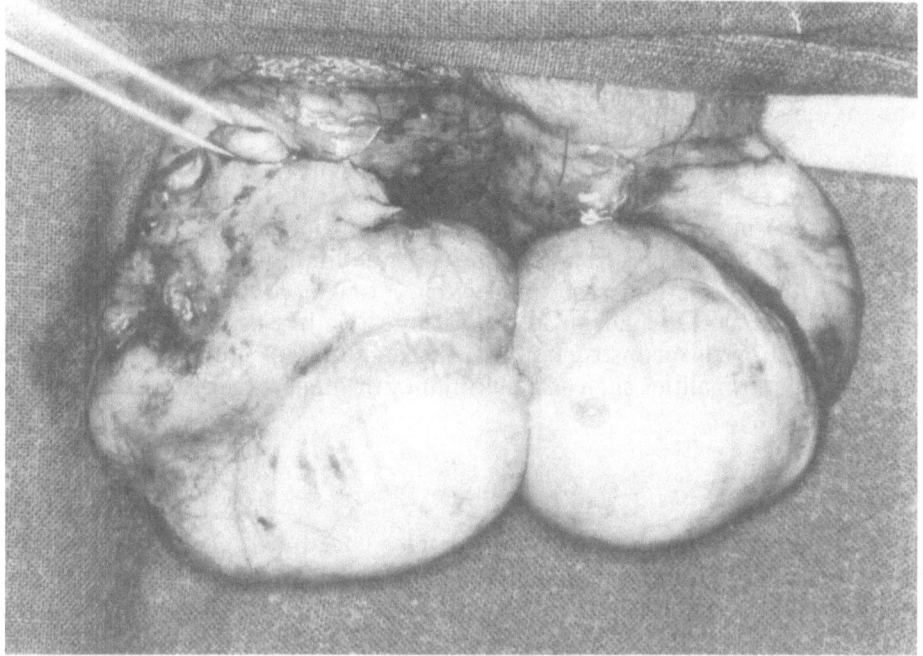

Figure 4.4 Unilateral caudal block: note the difference in the appearances of the obstructed right side (with tissue forcep) compared to the normal left side.

that it is clear, or to localise co-existing vasal blocks which may also require surgical correction.

After bilateral epididymo-vasostomies about 50% of patients in this category regain normal sperm counts, although this may take a year or more from the time of surgery.

A unilateral caudal block may be found not uncommonly. The appearances at exploratory scrototomy are characteristic and easy to recognise (Figure 4.4) by comparison with the opposite side.

Blocked vas

This occurs in its simplest form after vasectomy. Vasal blocks may also occur following infection, such as gonorrhoea, when they may co-exist with a caudal epididymal block, either on the same or on the other side. Ipsilateral caudal block is excluded by finding a good flow of milky fluid on incising the vas. The most common sites affected are the neck of the scrotum and the internal inguinal ring, where the vas changes direction sharply. Totally impenetrable blocks are occasionally encountered, which generally turn out to be tuberculous. The vas may also be obstructed following groin surgery such as hernia repair in infancy or childhood.

The level of the block may be defined by vasography (see below), which should also confirm patency of the vas beyond the block.

Absent vas

Bilateral absence of the vas was found in 17% of patients with azoospermia and normal FSH levels. If the seminal analysis indicates that this is the likely diagnosis (low pH, absent fructose) and the vas are impalpable, the patient need not be explored. Unilateral absence of the vas was found in 5% of the author's patients with azoospermia, associated with a variety of problems on the contralteral side such as testicular atrophy, post-infective blocks or other congenital anomalies. Surgical reconstruction was successful in 50% of cases. Associated urological abnormalities such as pelvic kidney or renal agenesis were also commonly present.

Ejaculatory duct

Obstruction at this level is rare, but examples have been seen with congenital anomalies such as Mullerian duct cysts or malformations of the ampullary part of the vas and seminal vesicle. Obstruction may also occur after excision of the rectum or following surgery for imperforate anus.

SURGICAL TECHNIQUE

Exploratory scrototomy

Surgery for male subfertility should always be done with good operating facilities and a general anaesthetic if possible. It is important to recognise that conditions which may be appropriate for simple vasectomy are not adequate for corrective or reconstructive surgery. Special facilities will be needed, such as fine instruments for microsurgical anastomoses, an operating microscope or magnifying spectacles, and equipment to allow X-rays to be taken on the operating table. A microscope will be required to examine fluid obtained from the epididymis or vas for the presence of spermatozoa.

These should be prepared in advance so that they are readily available at the time of surgery.

The scrotum is opened through a short midline incision, and the testicles are delivered. The tunica vaginalis is opened on both sides and the epididymes are examined for evidence of obstruction. If distended tubules are seen, the radiographer is notified that a vasogram will be required.

Whether or not there is evidence of obstruction, a testicular biopsy is taken next. A nick is made in the tunica albuginea, and a small piece of testicular tissue (about 2 mm diameter) is extruded and removed with scissors. The tissue is immediately fixed in Bouin's solution (**not** formalin), and may be sent for cytogenetic processing to study the meiotic chromosomes (Hendry *et al.*, 1975). The tunica albuginea is closed with a horizontal mattress suture of 3.0 chromic catgut. If the epididymes are empty, nothing further is done.

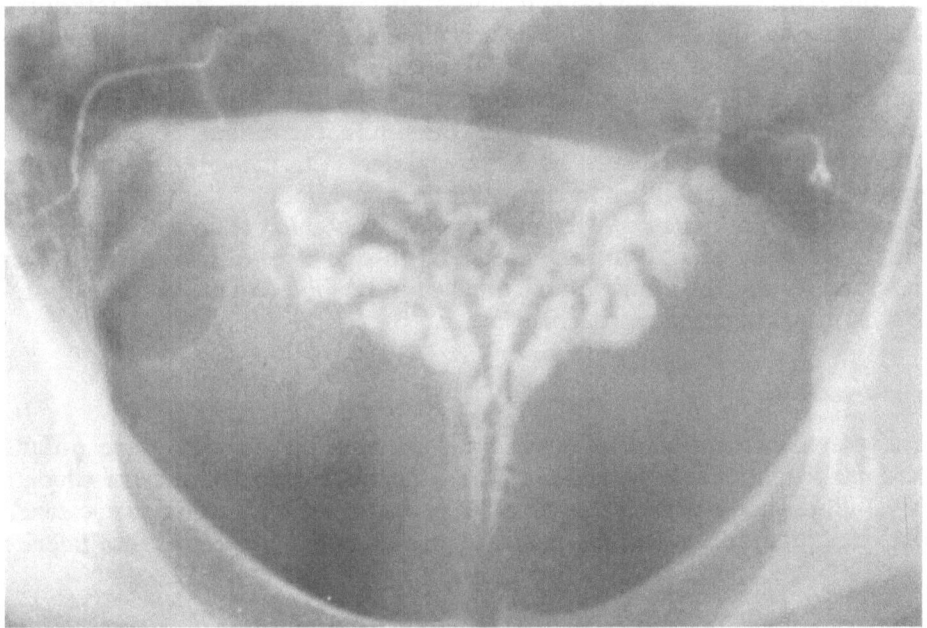

Figure 4.5 Normal vasogram. Note that the ejaculatory duct is clearly shown by directing the X-ray 20° down towards the feet - the so called 'open-pelvis' view.

If there is evidence of obstruction, vasography is done either by puncturing the vas with a fine needle, or by making a 0.5 cm longitudinal incision in the vas immediately adjacent to the lowest part of the epididymis that contains dilated tubules, and introducing a 2FG Portex polythene cannula. About 5 ml of radio-opaque contrast medium such as 25% Hypaque are injected up each side and an X-ray picture is taken (Figure 4.5).

Following the completion of reconstructive surgery (see below) the tunica vaginalis is closed on each side and the testes are returned to the scrotum. After applying a little antibiotic spray, the dartos layer is closed with continuous catgut, and the skin with a subcuticular nylon or Vicryl suture. The scrotum is wrapped in cotton wool, and placed in scrotal support which should remain dry and undisturbed for seven days.

Epididymo-vasostomy

After careful examination with the operating microscope or magnifying spectacles, the lowest part of the epididymis that contains dilated tubules is incised, and the fluid which runs out is examined immediately for the presence of sper-

and the fluid which runs out is examined immediately for the presence of spermatozoa. Once their presence has been confirmed, the incisions in the vas and
the epididymis, which should lie together without tension, are united. This can
be done most conveniently using double ended 6.0 Prolene, starting inferiorly.
The posterior edges are joined with a continuous suture and the anastomosis is
continued up to and around the critical superior end – the vasography cannula
may be left in while this part of the anastomosis is done. Once it is certain that
the lumen of the vas is not narrowed by the suture, the cannula is removed and
the anterior part of the anastomosis is completed. Alternatively, the epididymis
may be carefully mobilised by dissection from the body of the testis and then
transected. This can be repeated until free efflux of milky fluid is obtained, and
then the epididymis is anastomosed end-to-side or end-to-end to the vas
deferens. Ideally, the tubule exuding milky fluid is joined to the vas, mucosa-to-
mucosa using an operating microscope.

Vaso-vasostomy

For vasectomy reversal, an oblique incision is made on the lateral aspect of the
scrotum, so that it can be extended up to the inguinal region to obtain more length
of vas if this should prove necessary. The superior end is identified first, cleaned
of surrounding adhesions and mobilised enough to allow it to meet the inferior

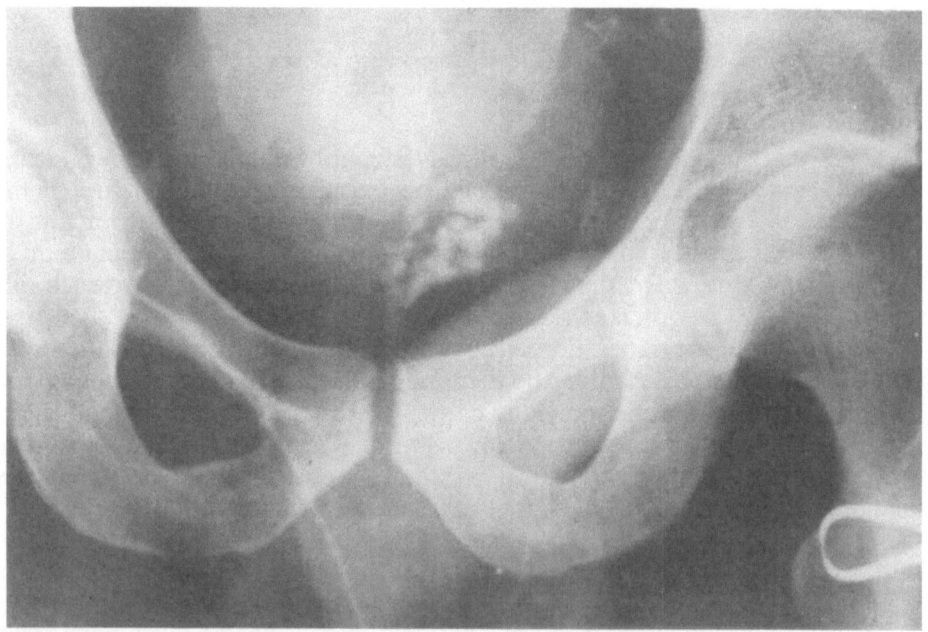

Figure 4.6 Vasogram showing a block at the internal inguinal ring on the right side, and a normal
left side.

end without tension. The inferior end is then identified and cleaned. Once the mobilisation is completed, a 0.5 cm linear incision is made in the inferior end of the vas just below the point of transection, and the tail of the epididymis is squeezed to express milky fluid from the vas. The superior end is similarly incised and the lumen defined with a fine nylon probe. The two ends are then overlapped and joined together by a side-to-side anastomosis using 6.0 Prolene and no splint.

Care should be taken to ensure that the anastomosis is as leak-proof as a vascular anastomosis, to prevent sperms from extravasating into the tissues and causing a sperm granuloma.

Alternatively, an end-to-end anastomosis may be done, but the fine bore of the lumen, and the disparity that often exists between the diameter of the upper and lower ends, requires a two layer microsurgical technique using the operating microscope if an accurate union is to be obtained.

If a vasal block is found in the patient with obstructive azoospermia in the course of exploratory scrototomy (Figure 4.6), it is generally best to make a counter incision in the groin to provide wide exposure of the vas so that the site of obstruction can be clearly defined with a view to reconstruction by vas-vasostomy. If there is a co-existing caudal epididymal block on the opposite testicle, or if that testis is atrophic, an alternative approach is trans-vaso-vasostomy. However, this has given rather disappointing results in the author's hands.

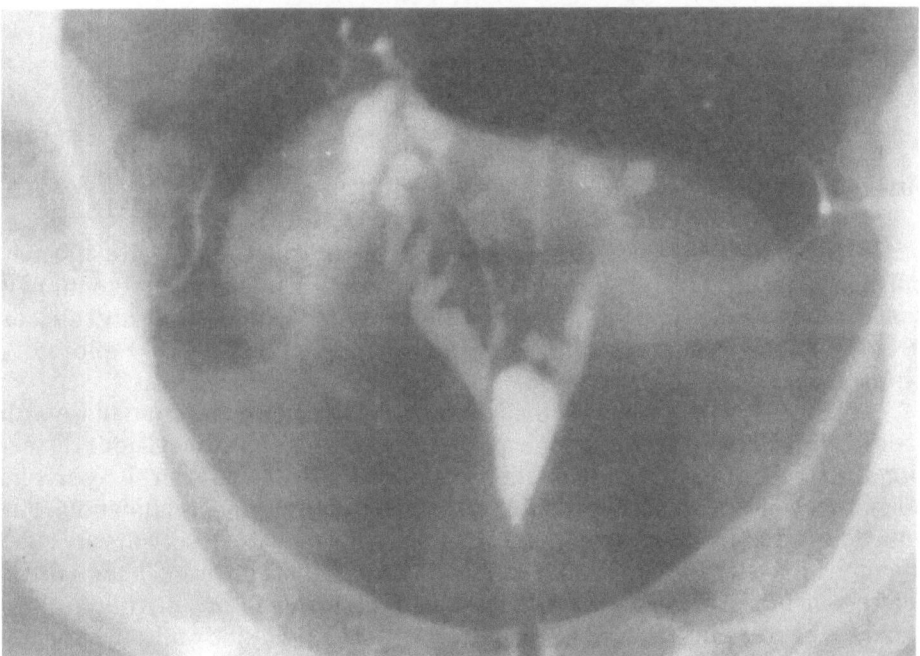

Figure 4.7 Vasogram showing ejaculatory duct cyst after transurethral incision: note that there is some dye in the bladder indicating that patency has been restored.

Ejaculatory duct obstruction

Surgical correction of these blocks is difficult, since the area is very inaccessible. However, endoscopic incision in the prostatic urethra can open into the ejaculatory duct, which may be more obvious if it has previously been filled with

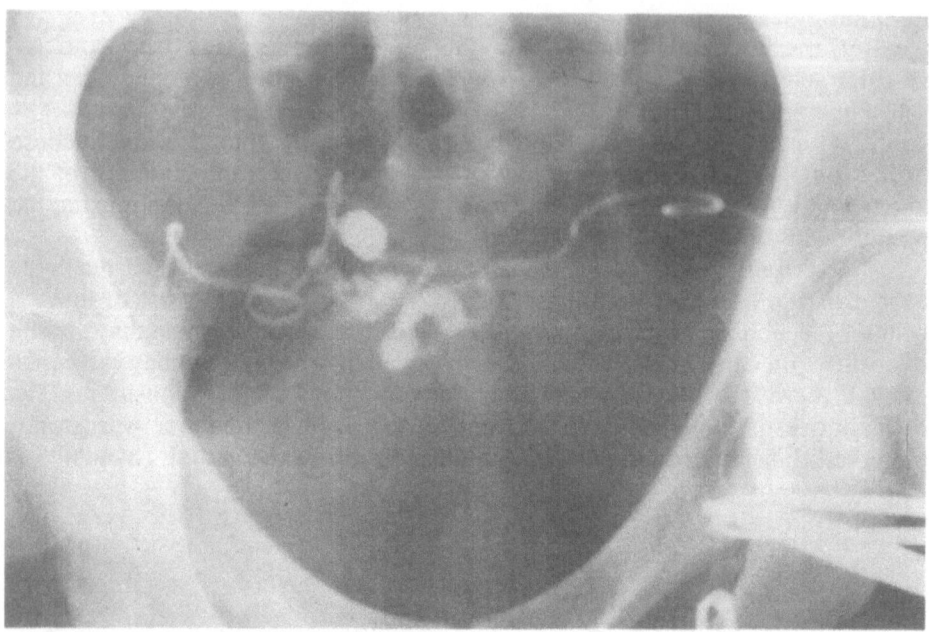

Figure 4.8 Ejaculatory duct obstruction following surgery for imperforate anus in childhood.

methylene blue at the time of vasography. Ejaculatory duct cyst (Figure 4.7) may bulge into the prostatic urethra and cause urinary difficulty or even retention: it can be easily recognised endoscopically and deroofed with the resectoscope, or deeply incised with the Colling's diathermy knife. Follow-up exploratory scrototomy and vasograms may be necessary if azoospermia persists.

Alternatively, patients with high vasal blocks (Figure 4.8), and those with failure of ejaculation due to paraplegia or following retroperitoneal node dissection, can be treated by implantation of specially designed sperm reservoirs (Figure 4.9), from which spermatozoa can be aspirated for insemination. The vasa deferentia are cannulated in the inguinal canal, and the reservoirs are sited under the deep fascia of the anterior abdominal wall just above and lateral to the internal inguinal ring. The reservoir has a selfsealing membrane in front to allow repeated needle puncture, and a rigid back plate and rigid side walls. In our early studies, motile spermatozoa have been recovered in 8 of 12 cases and two pregnancies produced (Brindley *et al.*, 1986).

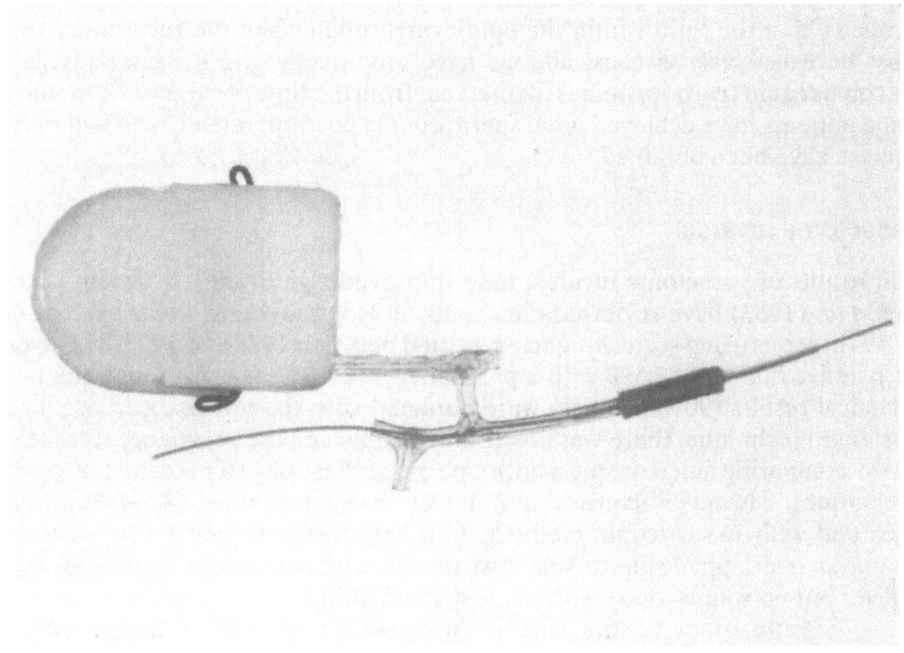

Figure 4.9 Sperm reservoirs for high vasal blocks or failure of ejaculation: the cannula is inserted into the vas deferens in the inguinal canal, and the reservoir lies subcutaneously: spermatozoa are obtained by needle puncture (Brindley *et al.*, 1986).

RESULTS OF SURGERY FOR TESTICULAR OBSTRUCTION

Obstructive azoospermia

In over one-third of our patients with obstructive azoospermia, acquired blocks of the cauda epididymes, vasa or ejaculatory duct were found, which were potentially suitable for surgical correction. Overall, spermatozoa returned to the ejaculate in 40% of these cases after surgery (excluding those lost to follow up, sperm counts of 20 million per ml or more were produced by 45% of 51 patients in these categories). Twenty-one per cent of wives with adequate follow up became pregnant: 17% of all patients in these categories, and 6.5% of the whole series of 168 patients (Hendry *et al.*, 1983). These figures may be compared with those of 51% patency and 21% pregnancy reported from 291 patients with adequate follow up by Schoysman (1982), and 55% patency and 29% pregnancy in 24 patients with a history of epididymitis (Dubin and Amelar, 1982).

On the other hand we had little success, apart from a few spermatozoa in the ejaculate, in patients with blocks in the caput epididymis. The association between chest disease and blocks in the caput epididymis (Young's syndrome) suggests that a defect in mucociliary function is the basic problem in this group of patients. Since the cilia are ultrastructurally and functionally normal in these patients (see above), we have assumed (until the precise underlying defect is defined), that the fluid within the epididymal tubules and the respiratory tree must be excessively viscous, and we have empirically given these patients a mucolytic agent (carbocysteine) for one year from the time of surgery. Since then, some patients have achieved good sperm counts post-operatively and two pregnancies have been obtained.

Vasectomy reversal

The results of vasectomy reversal have improved significantly in recent years. Cos *et al.* (1983) have reviewed the results of 943 vaso-vasostomies performed by 19 surgeons using six techniques, reported between 1978 and 1983. The overall patency rate was 82.5% with a pregnancy rate of 53.5%. Although the best technical results (90% patency) were obtained with the microscopic two layer unstented technique, there was no difference between the pregnancy rates (52–62%) comparing microscopic and loupe magnification, stented or unstented techniques. However, considerably lower pregnancy rates (41–44%) were recorded with macroscopic methods. Our experience supports this view, we favour an overlapped side-to-side anastomosis with continuous 60 prolene (see above) but no splints, done with loupe magnification.

Several other factors have been shown to have an influence on the likelihood of success. The findings of sperms in the fluid from the testicular end of the vas indicates a favourable prognosis, whereas the absence of such sperms is associated with an increasingly poor prognosis with lengthening time since vasectomy. The likelihood of regaining a normal sperm count falls to only 35% after more than 10 years (Silber, 1977). This may be due to the development of secondary changes in the epididymis; since vasectomy increases pressure in the testicular end of the vas which is transmitted to the epididymis. Rupture of the tubules in the epididymis may produce granulomata and secondary epididymal obstruction. Granuloma formation at the cut testicular end of the vas, however, is associated with reduction in dilatation of the vas and better quality vas fluid has been observed in the absence of such dilatation, possibly as a result of protection against back pressure (Silber, 1977). Vasectomy can also damage the nerves lying adjacent to the vas (Pabst *et al.*, 1979).

With a good surgical technique, vasectomy reversal should successfully restore a man's fertility in over 50% of cases. If the operation is unsuccessful – if sperms appear in the ejaculate only transiently or not at all – the scrotum should be re-explored: our results in 23 such cases are summarised in Table 4.2 (Royle and Hendry, 1985).

There appear to be four distinct causes of failure of vasectomy reversal. The commonest by far, which should be anticipated in about half of these patients, is due to stenosis or blockage of the previous vaso-vasostomy. It is known that spermatozoa tend to leak out of the anastomosis when vaso-vasostomy is done, and these may produce local granulomas (Hagan and Coffey, 1977). In 1977, Silber showed that carefully re-doing the vaso-vasostomies gave most satisfactory results with restoration of normal sperm counts, and a high incidence of pregnancy in the wives. Similarly, our success rate in this group was equivalent to that obtained on first doing vaso-vasostomies (Table 4.2).

The second most common cause is epididymal blockage, due to back pressure from the site of the vasectomy, leading to rupture of the epididymal tubules with local sperm granuloma formation within the epididymis. Excellent results can be obtained following epididymo-vasostomy in these cases, although restoration of normal sperm count takes rather longer than following vaso-vasostomy (Royle and Hendry, 1986).

Table 4.2 Results of re-exploration of scrotum in 23 patients who remained azoospermic after vasectomy reversal (from Royle and Hendry, 1985)

Category	Treatment	No.	Follow-up sperm counts			Pregnancies*
			0	< 20	> 20	
1 Blocked vas	Redo vas-vas	12	1	3	7	5/8 (62%)
2 Epididymal block	Ep-vas	4	1		3	2/4 (50%)
3 Antisperm antibodies (1024)	Surgery + prednisolone	7	1	3	3	0/7
						7/19 (37%)

(* trying for 6 months or more)

The problem of the patient who develops very high antisperm antibody response to his vasectomy continues to defy successful treatment. In our previous studies (Parslow et al., 1983) we showed that pregnancy was possible despite high antisperm antibody titres, but we have defined a small sub-population in whom, despite re-exploration of the scrotum and Prednisolone therapy (Hendry et al., 1986), restoration of fertility does not seem to be possible, apparently due to the immunological response to the spermatozoa. This problem continues to present a significant therapeutic challenge (see Chapter 6).

Finally, spermatogenesis may have ceased. However, our studies, and those of Bagshaw et al., (1980), showed by testicular biopsy that significant impairment of spermatogenesis following vasectomy is in fact extremely uncommon. Nevertheless, the possibility should be considered amongst the population of patients, many of whom are entering middle life at the time that this surgery is carried out.

Unilateral testicular obstruction

Unilateral obstruction may be difficult to diagnose. We first studied 32 subfertile males with sperms in the ejaculate and unilateral testicular obstruction (Hendry *et al.*, 1982): the past medical history gave relevant information in 84% and useful findings were made on clinical examination in a few. Since then, this experience has been extended to 80 spontaneously infertile males, in whom the presence of unilateral testicular obstruction has been confirmed by exploratory

Table 4.3 Sites and probable causes of unilateral obstruction in 80 subfertile males. (from Hendry, 1986)

	Post-infective	Surgery/injury	Congenital	Cause unknown
Upper epididymis		5		6
Tail of epididymis	25	6		9
Vas deferens	8	12	4	
Ejaculatory duct	1	2	1	1
Total	34	25	5	16

Table 4.4 Pregnancies produced/number treated in 60 patients with adequate follow up related to initial sperm counts and surgical treatment. (from Hendry, 1986)

Surgical treatment	Initial sperm count M/ml			
	< 5	6–20	> 20	Totals
Ep-vas	7/18	1/10	2/5	10/33 (30%)
Vas-vas	2/5		1/1	3/6 (50%)
Orchidectomy	1/2	0/2	1/6	2/10 (20%)
None (steroids)	2/5	1/2	1/4	4/11 (36%)
Total	12/30 (40%)	2/14 (14%)	5/16 (31%)	19/60 (32%)

scrototomy (Hendry, 1986). Half of these patients had severe oligozoospermia with sperm counts of less than 5 million per ml even though testicular biopsies showed adequate spermatogenesis, and despite the presence of an unobstructedcontralateral testis. The sperm count was normal (greater than 20 million per ml) in only 21. Sixty one patients (75%) had serum antisperm antibodies, presumably provoked by the testicular obstruction. The most common sites of obstruction were at the tail of the epididymis, or in the vas deferens (Table 4.3).

Corrective surgery was done by epididymo-vasotomy or vaso-vasotomy whenever possible, but in 11 cases when repair was impossible the obstucted testis was removed and replaced with a prosthesis. Steroid treatment for antisperm antibodies was given when appropriate. One third of 60 patients with adequate follow-up successfully impregnated their female partners, with paradoxically, the best results occurring in 30 men who started with sperm counts of less than 5 million per ml, 12 (40%) of whom were successful Table 4.4).

Clinical history, physical examination and the presence of antisperm antibodies, can suggest the possibility of unilateral testicular obstruction, but confirmation of the diagnosis requires exploratiory scrototomy. Unilateral obstruction, a correctable cause of infertility, should be recognised and treated.

SUMMARY AND CONCLUSIONS

The diagnosis and correction of testicular obstruction is clearly an integral part of the treatment of an infertile male. However, the urologist must look beyond the actual blockage, to the pathological condition causing it, and to its immunological consequences, if the results of such treatment are to improve.

References

Bagshaw, H.A., Masters, J.R.W. and Pryor, J.P. (1980). Factors influencing the outcome of vasectomy reversal. *Br. J. Urol.*, **52**, 57–60

Brindley, G.S., Scott, G.I. and Hendry, W.F. (1986). Vas cannulation with implanted sperm-reservoirs for obstructive azoospermia or ejaculatory failure. *Br. J. Urol.*, **58**, 721–3

Cos, L.R., Valvo, J.R., Davis, R.S. and Cockett, A.J.K. (1983). Vasovasostomy: current state of the art. *Urol.*, **22**, 567–75

Dubin, L. and Amelar, R.D. (1982). Epididymovasostomy. In Garcia, C.R., Mastroianni, L., Amelar, R.D. and Dubin, L. (eds.) *Current Therapy of Infertility*. pp. 77–9. (Trenton, B.C. Decker) Hagan, K.F. and Coffey, D.S. (1977). The adverse effects of sperm during vasovasostomy. *J. Urol.*, **118**, 269–273

Handelsman, D.J., Conway, A.J., Boylan, L.M. and Turtle, J.R. (1984). Young's syndrome: obstructive azoospermia and chronic sinopulmonary infections. *N.Engl. J. Med.*, **310**, 3–9

Hendry, W.F. (1986). The clinical significance of unilateral testicular obstruction in subfertile males. *Br. J. Urol.*, **58**, 709–14

Hendry, W.F., Polani, P.E., Pugh, R.C.B., Sommerville, I.F. and Wallace, D.M. (1975). 200 infertile males: correlation of chromosome, histological, endocrine and clinical studies. *Br. J. Urol.*, **47**, 899–908

Hendry, W.F., Knight, R.K., Whitfield, H.N. *et al.* (1978). Obstructive azoospermia: respiratory function tests, electron microscopy and the results of surgery. *Br. J. Urol.*, **50**, 598–604

Hendry, W.F., Parslow, J.M., Stedronska, J. and Wallace, D.M.A. (1982). The diagnosis of unilateral testicular obstruction in subfertile males. *Br. J. Urol.*, **54**, 774–9

Hendry, W.F., Parslow, J.M. and Stedronska, J. (1983). Exploratory scrototomy in 168 azoospermic males. *Br. J. Urol.*, **55**, 785–91

Hendry, W.F., Treehuba, K., Hughes, L., Stedronska, J., Parslow, J.M, Wass, J.A.H. and Besser, G.M. (1986). Cyclic prednisolone therapy for male infertility associated with antibodies to spermatozoa. *Fertil. Steril.*, **45**, 249–254

Neville, E., Brewis, R., Yeates, W.K. and Burridge, A. (1983). Respiratory tract disease and obstructive azoospermia. *Thorax*, **38**, 929–33

Pabst, R., Martin, O. and Lippert, H. (1979). Is the low fertility rate after vasovasostomy caused by nerve resection during vasectomy? *Fertil. Steril.*, **31**, 316–20

Parslow, J.M., Royle, M.G., Kingscott, M.M.B., Wallace, D.M.A. and Hendry, W.F. (1983). The effects of sperm antibodies on fertility after vasectomy reversal. *Am. J. Reprod. Immunol.*, **3**, 28–31

Pavia, D., Agnew, J.E., Bateman, J.R.M., Sheahan, N.F., Knight, R.K., Hendry, W.F. and Clarke, S.W. (1981). Lung microciliary clearance in patients with Young's syndrome. *Chest*, **80**, supplement 892–95

Royle, M.G. and Hendry, W.F. (1985). Why does vasectomy reversal fail? *Br. J. Urol.*, **57**, 780–3

Rutland, J. and Cole, P.J. (1980). Non-invasive sampling of nasal cilia for measurement of beat frequency and study of ultrastructure. *Lancet*, **2**, 564–5

Schoysman, R. (1982). Epididymal causes of male infertility: pathogenesis and management. In White, R. de V. (ed.) *Aspect of Male Infertility*. pp. 233–49. (Baltimore: Williams and Wilkins)

Silber, S.J. (1977). Microscopic vasectomy reversal. *Fertil. Steril.*, **28**, 1191–1202

Young, D. (1970). Surgical treatment of male infertility. *J. Reprod. Fertil.*, **23**, 541–2

DISCUSSION

Question: Do you perform testicular biopsies routinely when doing a vasovasostomy?

Hendry: No. Spermatogenesis is normal post vasectomy. We would only perform a testicular biopsy on a repeat vasovasostomy.

Question: Why in unilateral absence of vas do you have azoospermia?

Hendry: Usually because something has happened on the other side.

Question: Are immunological problems created by performing testicular biopsies?

Hendry: No. Studies have been performed using antisperm antibodies before and after.

Question: What is your experience of the time interval between performing the vasovasostomy and the establishment of a normal sperm count and pregnancy?

Hendry: On average 6-12 months

Question: Is 'Young's Syndrome' the same as immotile cilia syndrome?

Hendry: No. In Young's Syndrome cilia move normally. The differential diagnosis is made by – vasa both sides, cilia moving and azoospermia.

Question: Do you need azoospermia for Young's Syndrome?

Hendry: No. The patient may present with deteriorating sperm count.

Question: How reliable is the impression of distended tubules for obstruction?

Hendry: Very reliable. When using magnifying glasses the situation is obvious. If no distended tubules are seen then there is no obstruction unless the obstruction is at the region of the rete testis.

Question: Is there any data on the relationship between site of epididymo-vasostomy and sperm numbers.

Hendry: Yes. The higher up the reanastomosis the lower the chance of sperm being present in the ejaculate.

5
VARICOCELE AND ITS TREATMENT

F.H. Comhaire

INTRODUCTION

Varicocele is present in 8–18% of all adolescent men; this condition therefore can hardly be considered a disease (Handelsman et al., 1984). However, presumably one out of five men with varicocele will suffer from a complication of this condition, such as impaired fertility, decreased androgen secretion and sexual inadequacy (Comhaire and Vermeulen, 1975), or local discomfort. Besides, varicocele seems to promote the occurrence of male accessory gland infection and autoimmunity against spermatozoa (Comhaire et al., 1987).

In spite of a few reports to the contrary, the causal link between varicocele and subfertility is generally accepted. The degree of fertility disturbance appears to be independent of the volume of the varicocele (Etriby et al., 1967). Impairment of semen quality may occur later in reproductive life, resulting in secondary sterility.

PHYSIOPATHOLOGY

Varicocele is due to reflux of renal and adrenal blood into the internal spermatic vein and pampiniform plexus. This refluxing blood contains an increased concentration of norepinephrine (Comhaire and Vermeulen, 1974). After counter current exchange in the pampiniform plexus, norepinephrine causes arteriolar constriction which results in decreased blood supply to the testis. This phenomenon has been documented in studies of testicular perfusion using technetium-99m pertechnetate as a tracer (Comhaire et al., 1984). Testicular arterial perfusion usually normalizes rapidly after interruption of reflux, which results in progressive improvement of semen quality. Patients not presenting normalization of testicular perfusion do not seem to benefit from treatment.

The physiopathological mechanism described above is probably not the only one responsible for testicular damage, since it can be documented in only 50% of patients. Among other factors which may interfere, the most commonly cited are increased hydrostatic pressure and impaired fluid handling (Harrison et al., 1983), as well as increased testicular temperature (Zorgniotti and Mac-Leod, 1973). Besides, there is as yet no satisfactory explanation for the fact that varicocele often does not, and only sometimes does, impair testicular-epididymal function.

DIAGNOSIS

Reflux into the internal spermatic vein, together with impairment of testicular function may also occur in the absence of palpable dilatation of the scrotal pampiniform plexus. The diagnosis of these 'subclinical varicoceles' can be made with several methods. Scanning of the scrotum after technetium-99m pertechnetate injection detects blood stasis in the pampiniform plexus and may depict a non-radiological angiogram (Freund *et al.*, 1980). In the absence of blood stasis, particularly in patients without distension of the pampiniform plexus, the technetium scan will miss the diagnosis (Comhaire *et al.*, 1982).

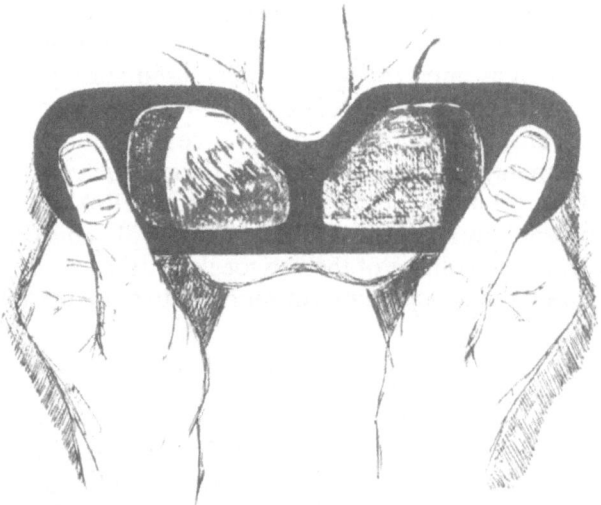

Figure 5.1 Contact thermography for varicocele diagnosis by means of VARICOSCREEN® (Amsaten Corp., Keistraat, 139, B-9720 De Pinte, Belgium).

Since the temperature of the scrotal skin in normal men is 33°C or less, and since in varicocele warm blood refluxes into the pampiniform plexus, reflux will result in an increased temperature of the scrotal skin overlying the pampiniform plexus (Kormano *et al.*, 1970). Such zones of increased temperatures can be detected by scrotal thermography. Both telethermography and contact thermography, in particular making use of flexible Varicoscreens (Figure 5.1), are indeed excellent methods for the detection of both clinical and subclinical varicoceles (World Health Organization, 1985).

The Doppler method allows for the directional analysis of blood flow. This method can be applied successfully to detect inversion of blood flow in the internal spermatic vein and paminiform plexus of patients with varicocele.

However, the technique is more delicate and subject to misinterpretation than thermography. Doppler flow measurement should be considered a useful completion of thermographic examination.

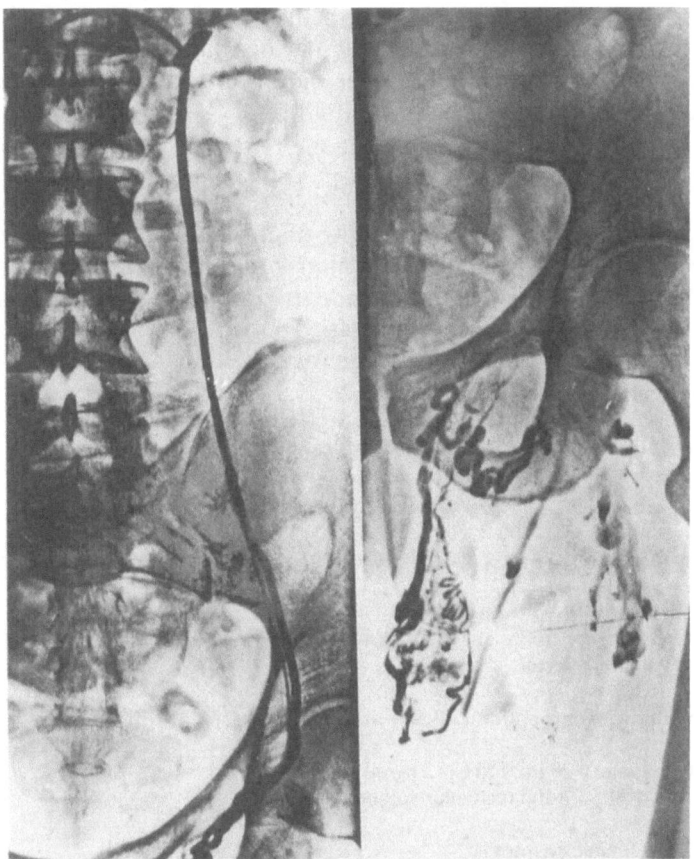

Figure 5.2 Retrograde venography of the left internal spermatic vein in a patient with varicocele (courtesy M. Kunnen, Dept. Radiology).

The presence of reflux in the internal spermatic vein can be visualised radiologically by retrograde venography from the renal vein (Figure 5.2). In addition, retrograde venography depicts the pathway taken by the refluxing blood and discloses the exact anatomy of the internal spermatic venous complex, which commonly is greatly aberrant (Comhaire *et al.*, 1981; Bigot *et al.*, 1982). Retrograde venography of the right internal spermatic vein has proved reflux to be bilateral in one third of cases.

TREATMENT OF VARICOCELE

Treatment of varicocele is classically surgical (Ivanissivich, 1924; Bernardi, 1942; Dubin and Amelar, 1977). The incision should be made a few centimetres cranially of the left groin and all spermatic venous branches allowing reflux should be ligated and transsected just cranially of the internal inguinal ring. The fact that, in doing so, the testicular artery may be interrupted as well, seems to do no harm to the testis, provided that the defferential and cremasteric arteries are left unaltered (Wallijn and Desmet, 1978).

TREATMENT RESULTS

The cumulative pregnancy rate after transcatheter embolization of the internal spermatic vein using a tissue adhesive in men with subnormal semen is shown in Figure 5.3. Several factors were found to determine the fertility after varicocele treatment (Table 5.1). The success rate varies between 8 and 80% depending on total testicular volume, clinical stage of the varicocele and serum FSH concentration (Figure 5.4).

Table 5.1 Probability of success after varicocele treatment

High probability of conception (> 50% overall success rate

Grade II-III varicocele + FSH < 2 ng/ml	80%
Secondary infertility	78%
No other factors in the man or woman	65%
Motile sperm count before treatment > 2 mill/ml	62%
Total testicular volume > 28 ml	60%

Moderate probability of conception (20–50% overall success rate)

Total testicular volume > 28 ml, FSH > 2 ng/ml	40%
Grade II–III varicocele + total testicular volume > 28 ml	30%
Other factor in the female partner	30%
Motile sperm count before treatment < 0.5 mill/ml	30%

Poor probability of conception (< 20% overall success rate)

Simultaneous male accessory gland infection	12%
Grade I or subclinical varicocele + total testicular volume < 28 ml	8%
Serum FSH > 6 ng/ml	0%
Simultaneous sperm antibodies	0%

The observed pregnancy rate after treatment of 3.9% per cycle is clearly higher than the spontaneous pregnancy rate of couples who are waiting to be treated. The latter is 0.6% per cycle, since only one pregnancy occured in 35 couples followed during a total of 172 couple-months before treatment.

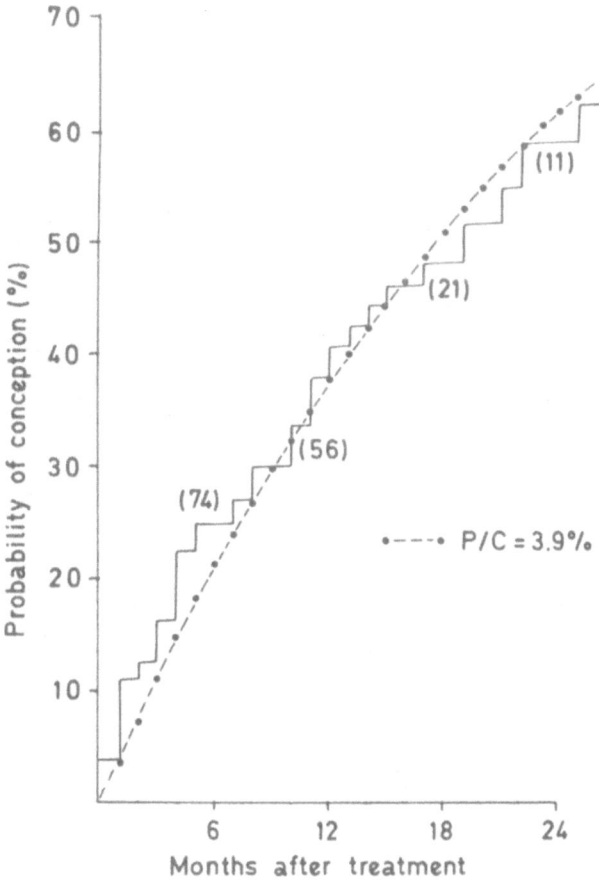

Figure 5.3 Cumulative pregnancy rate after varicocele treatment by transcatheter embolization with a tissue adhesive.

Recently, treatment of varicocele by transcatheter sclerosis (Lima *et al.*, 1978) or embolization with tissue adhesive (Kunnen, 1980) has been introduced in several clinics. Up to now, over 750 patients have been treated with this method in our centre. The non-surgical approach has the advantage of requiring neither general anaesthesia nor hospitalization. Transcatheter obliteration is performed in immediate sequence to retrograde venography, using the same set of catheters. The result of treatment can be evaluated by means of control venography during the same session.

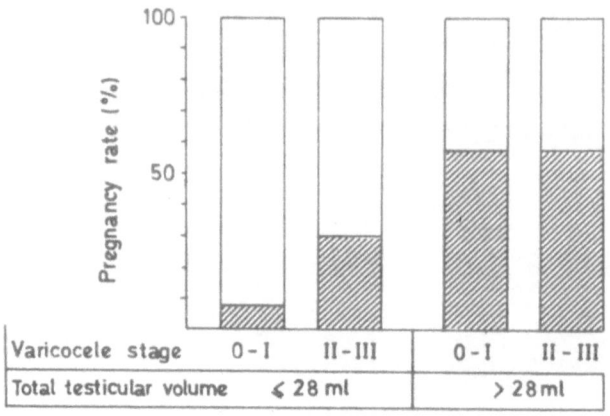

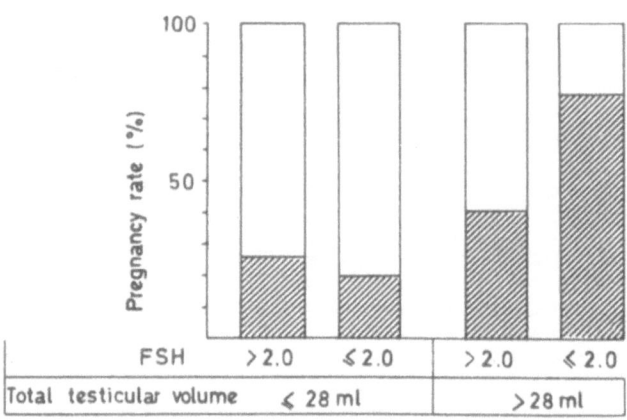

Figure 5.4 Overall success rate after varicocele embolization related to varicocele stage, total testicular volume and serum FSH concentration (in ng/ml) (From Cromhaire & Kunnen, 1985, by permission).

CONCLUSION

Varicocele is a common anatomical condition which may deteriorate into a disease interfering with such vital functions as reproduction and sexual adequacy. It can be estimated that about 0.5% of all men remain sterile due to varicocele disease, in spite of all attempts of treatment. It remains an open question whether treatment of varicocele at the beginning of puberty may prevent the deterioration of testicular function.

Since the introduction of a highly successful non-surgical method to cure varicocele, prophylactic treatment may be appropriate.

Whereas the majority of studies suggest a beneficial effect of varicocele treatment, others cast doubt on its effectiveness. Although there is ample evidence to suggest a favourable effect of varicocele treatment, there is still need for a carefully controlled prospective study to unequivocally prove the therapeutic effect. Whilst awaiting the result of such studies patients should be treated for their varicocele.

ACKNOWLEDGEMENTS

This work was supported by the World Health Organisation, Special Programme of Research, Development and Research Training in Human Reproduction.

References

Bernardi, R. (1942). New incision for therapy of varicocele: semeilogic and surgical concepts. *Sem. Med.*, **2**, 165

Bigot, J.M., Barrett, F. and Helenon, C. (1982). Phlebography of the right spermatic vein in varicocele. In Jecht, E.W. and Zeitler, E. (eds.) *Varicocele and Male Infertility. Recent Advances in Diagnosis and Therapy.* pp. 59–67. (Berlin: Springer Verlag)

Comhaire, F.H. (1986). Varicocele and its role in male infertility. In *Oxford Reviews of Reproductive Biology*, Vol 8, pp. 165–213

Comhaire, F. and Kunnen, M. (1985). Factors affecting the probability of conception after treatment of subfertile men with varicocele by transcatheter embolization with Bucrylate (R). *Fertil. Steril.*, **43**, 781

Comhaire, F., Kunnen, M. and Hahoum, C. (1981). Radiological anatomy of the internal spermatic vein(s) in 200 retrograde venograms. *Int. J. Androl.*, **4**, 379

Comhaire, F., Kunnen, M and Simons, M. (1984). Physiopathology of testicular dysfunction in varicocele: does varicocele exist without reflux in the internal spermatic vein? In Glezermen, M. and Jecht, E.W (eds.) pp. 88–96. (Berlin: Springer Verlag)

Comhaire, F., Kunnen, M., Vandeweghe, M. and Simons, M. (1982). Comparison between different methods for the diagnosis of varicocele. In Jecht, E.W. and Zeitler, E. (eds.) *Varicocele and Male Infertility. Recent Advances in Diagnosis and Therapy.* pp. 88–96. (Berlin: Springer Verlag)

Comhaire, F., Rowe, P. and Farley, T. (1987). Towards more objectivity in the management of male infertility. *Int. J. Androl.*, Suppl. 7, p. 1–53

Comhaire, F. and Vermeulen, A. (1974). Varicocele sterility: Cortisol and cathecholamines. *Fertil. Steril.*, **25**, 88

Comhaire, F. and Vermeulen, A. (1975). Plasma testosterone in patients with varicocele and sexual inadequacy. *J. Clin. Endocr. Metab.*, **40**, 824

Dubin, L. and Amelar, R.D. (1977). Varicocele and results of varicocelectomy in selected subfertile men with varicocele. *Fertil. Steril.*, **21**, 606

Etriby, A., Girgis, S.M., Hefnawy, H. and Ibrahim, A.A. (1967). Testicular changes in subfertile males with varicocele. *Fertil. Steril.*, **18**, 666

Freund, J., Handelsman, D.J., Conway, G.J. and Morris, J.G. (1980). Detection of varicocele by radionuclide blood-pool scanning. *Radiology*, **137**, 227

Handelsman, D.J., Conway, A.J., Doylan, L.M. and Turtle, J.R. (1984). Testicular function in potential sperm donors: normal ranges and the effects of smoking and varicocele. *Int. J. Androl.*, 7, 369

Harrison, R.M., Lewis, R.W. and Roberts, J.A. (1983). Testicular blood flow and fluid dynamics in monkeys with surgically induced varicoceles. *J. Androl.*, 4, 256

Ivanessivich, O. (1924). Las venas espermaticas del lazo izquierdo. Estado en 40 desecciones cadavericas y en 20 operationes por hernia y varicocele. *Sem. Med.*, 1, 1191

Kormano, M., Kahanpaa, K., Svinhufvud, U. and Tahti, E. (1970). Thermography of varicocele. *Fertil. Steril.*, 21, 558

Kunnen, M. (1980). Neue Technik zun Embolisation der Vena spermatica interna: intravenoser Gewebekleber. *Fortschr. Rontgenstr.*, 133, 625

Lima, S.S., Castro, M.P. and Costa, O. (1978). A new method for the treatment of varicocele. *Andrologia*, 10, 103

Wallijn, E. and Desmet, R. (1978). Hydrocele: a frequently overlooked complication after high ligation of the spermatic vein for varicocele. *Int. J. Androl.*, 1, 411

World Health Organisation (1985). Comparison among different methods for the diagnosis of varicocele. *Fertil. Steril.*, 43, 575

Zorgniotti, A.W. and MacLeod, J. (1973). Studies in temperature, human semen quality and varicocele. *Fertil. Steril.*, 24, 854

DISCUSSION

Question: It has been suggested that men with an incidentally discovered varicocele should be investigated. As a Urologist I disagree with this – can you comment?

Comhaire: Whether it makes sense to perform 'prophylactic' treatment of incidentally detected varicocele in young adolescents will depend on the risk/benefit ratio of treatment. Varicocele usually develops at puberty and has been shown to impair testicular (tubular) histology at this early age. On the other hand, a substantial proportion of fertile men have varicocele, proving that varicocele does not always impair fertility. Epidemiological data on the risk of a young varicocele carrier to develop infertility or to remain infertile after varcicocele treatment for subfertility, are lacking. Indirect evidence permits to calculate that 10–15% of adolescents with varicocele will have fertility problems. Since fertility is restored by treatment in half these cases, 5–7% will remain permanently sterile. Hence, the risk of varicocele to cause permanent infertility can be estimated around 5–7%. The risk of varicocele treatment depends on the method used. Whereas the complication rate of surgery is 5–10% (commonly hydrocele, rarely testicular atrophy), that of transcatheter embolization is less than 0.5% in our hands (usually minor complications of the Seldinger catheterization). Considering the favourable risk/benefit ratio of the latter treatment, prophylactic embolization might be advocated on theoretical grounds.

In addition, men with varicocele have a significantly increased risk to develop accessory gland infection as well as immunological factors. Both these elements unfavourably influence fertility, adding to my argument for prophylactic treatment. Evidently, prospective studies should be carried out before this policy is generally sustained.

Question: Are you suggesting that all men of 16 who have a varicocele should be treated?

Comhaire: Yes, provided good facilities are available to carry out the non-surgical treatment which I have described.

Question: Is there a time related deterioration in men with varicocele?

Comhaire: Yes. Several studies have shown time related deterioration of Leydig cell function and of testosterone response to hCG stimulation. As far as fertility is concerned available evidence is scant but suggestive.

6
IMMUNOLOGICAL ASPECTS OF MALE INFERTILITY

W.F. Hendry

very male and female partner in an infertile marriage should be fully tested for antisperm antibodies. However, this would put a strain on laboratory services and inevitably produce problems with false positive results. It is probably not necessary, provided that the mode of action of antisperm antibodies is remembered, and simple screening tests are understood.

SEMINAL ANALYSIS AND POST-COITAL TEST

Taken together, these two basic tests exclude immunological infertility, provided both are normal. A normal sperm count should exceed 20 m/ml, with more than 40% moving actively within three hours of production in a volume of at least 1.5 ml (Macleod, 1951; Macleod and Gold, 1951). However, the spermatozoa must be able to produce an adequate post coital test (PCT) in normal ovulatory cervical mucus – this is usually defined as more than five motile sperms per high power field (Santomauro et al., 1972).

The co-existence of a normal sperm count and a persistently poor PCT suggests the possible existence of antisperm antibodies, and these commonly occur in the husband. Kremer et al., (1978a) investigated 30 couples with persistently poor PCT due to antisperm antibodies and found that the antibodies were present in the husband in 25, and in the wife in only five cases. The partner with the antibodies can be identified by direct testing for antisperm antibodies and confirmed by sperm cervical mucus contact (SCMC) testing (see below) using donor sperms and mucus as controls. The presence of agglutination of sperms in a semen specimen does not, by itself, indicate the presence of antibodies. If the man has a low sperm count, antisperm antibody testing should form part of the diagnostic work up, and must always be included in the evaluation of azoospermia.

There remains the possibility that the PCT might be poor for other reasons, or the results may not be available at the time that the husband's fertility status is under review. Since he always produces a semen specimen for analysis, a direct antibody test on the patient's spermatozoa is obviously most useful as a screening test. The mixed erythrocyte–spermatozoa antiglobulin reaction (MAR) test is ideal for this purpose.

MIXED ERYTHROCTYE–SPERMATOZOA ANTIGLOBULIN REACTION (MAR TEST)

This simple and rapid screening test was introduced by Jager *et al.* (1978). The test is based on the formation of motile mixed agglutinates between erythrocytes sensitised with incomplete anti-Rh antibodies. After mixing one drop of the sensitised red cells with one drop of patient's semen and one drop of anti-human IgG antiserum (Behring), the result is read within 10 minutes: **negative, doubtful** less than 10% of motile spermatozoa incorporated in mixed agglutinates: **positive** 10–90% and **strongly positive** over 90% of motile sperms caught in clumps. Agglutination of the red cells serves as an internal control. We evaluated this test with semen samples from the male partners of infertile marriages, and a satisfactory reaction was obtained with 86% of specimens. The test was unsatisfactory in the remainder because of severely abnormal sperm count of very low motility. It was concluded that this test was a very useful addition to routine semen analysis, but that positive results should be further assessed by accurate estimation of antibody titres before recommending treatment (Stedronska and Hendry, 1983).

ANTISPERM ANTIBODY TEST FOR SERUM OR SEMINAL PLAMSA

The technical details of the various tests have been defined by a WHO workshop (Rose *et al.*, 1976), and the results of an international comparative study in men and women were reported by the WHO Reference Bank for Reproductive Immunology (1977). The gelatin agglutination test (GAT) and sperm immobilisation test (SIT) have given reliable and reproducible results in men (Hendry *et al.*, 1977; Husted, 1975). The tray agglutination test (TAT) is particularly useful because it can be done on small quantities of genital secretions, and it is probably the best test for detecting relatively low titres of antibodies in females (Friberg, 1974). We have stopped doing immunofluorescent studies, as we found that over 30% of patients showed a positive result irrespective of whether they had antisperm antibodies detectable by other means or not, and because there was no correlation with impaired sperm penetration of cervical mucus. Similarly it appears that antibodies detected by enzyme linked immunosorbent assay (ELISA) are not the same as those detected by tray agglutination test and these tests are not recommended for evaluation of the subfertile couple (Stedronska–Clarke *et al.*, 1987).

SPERM CERVICAL MUCUS CONTACT (SCMC) TEST

By studying directly the reaction between spermatozoa and the new environment in which they must survive and make forward progression, this test provides the reference point against which all other observations should be checked. If this simple test is done with fertile donor sperms and cervical mucus as controls, ('Crossed Hostility Test'), it gives positive evidence as to which partner is likely to have the antibodies, and provides fundamental confirmation that the results obtained by other tests are reflected by significant interference with sperm activity.

A positive reaction is shown by the change from progressive movement to a characteristic non-progressive 'shaking' movement. Kremer *et al.* (1978b) showed that a positive 'shaking phenomenon' is dependent upon the presence of immunoglobulin A on the spermatozoa.

EFFECTS OF ANTISPERM ANTIBODIES

Antisperm antibodies can occur in men with normal or low sperm counts, and it is evident that these antibodies can interfere with the fertilising capacity of the spermatozoa by preventing them from penetrating cervical mucus. However, it is difficult to be sure exactly what titre of agglutinating antibodies is required to produce relative or complete sterility. Rumke *et al.* (1974) studied this question by following men who had normal sperm counts and positive serum agglutination tests for 10 years. Almost half of the men with serum titres of less than 32 produced pregnancies, whereas there was a progressive decline in fertility as the antibody titre rose above this level. A serum titre of 32 is therefore generally accepted as the minimum titre for significance in men, although it should be noted that a few spontaneous pregnancies should be anticipated, produced by men with titres above this level. Fjallbrant (1968) compared fertile and sterile men, and showed a strong negative correlation between the concentration of antibodies and the ability of sperms to penetrate ovulatory cervical mucus, and observed that the interrelation between sperm penetration ability and subsequent fertility was very good.

Estimates of the incidence of antisperm antibodies in men have varied a little. Taking a dilution of 1 in 32 as the limit of significance for serum agglutination titres, the incidence of antisperm antibodies in fertile men presenting for vasectomy was 2%, compared with 13.4% in subfertile men (Halim and Antoniou, 1973). We found 8.5% positive in 591 subfertile men (Hendry *et al.*, 1977). In 21 of 22 couples tested, spermatozoa from husbands with antisperm antibodies (GAT titre / 32) could not penetrate cervical mucus – neither their wives' nor fertile donors' – whereas fertile donor sperms showed good penetration of both specimens of mucus (Morgan *et al.*, 1977). This demonstrated that the phenomenon commonly known as 'cervical hostility' could often be due to antisperm antibodies in the husband. The one exception out of the 22 couples was a man with serum antisperm antibodies following reversal of vasectomy, whose sperms showed good mucus penetration; he subsequently impregnated his wife without further treatment – the odd-man-out who will be considered in more detail later.

The distinction between antisperm antibodies in serum (IgG) and in seminal plasma (IgA) is important because they do not always occur together, and because a blood test can only detect serum antibodies whereas it is the seminal plasma antibody which interferes directly with fertility. Rumke (1978) has shown that the proportion of naturally subfertile men who have seminal plasma antibodies rises in a linear manner once the serum antibody titre exceeds 32. In contrast, few vasectomised men develop seminal plasma antibodies until the serum titre is very high (≥ 512), and even after reversal the proportion with such antibodies is less than in spontaneously infertile men (Figure 6.1).

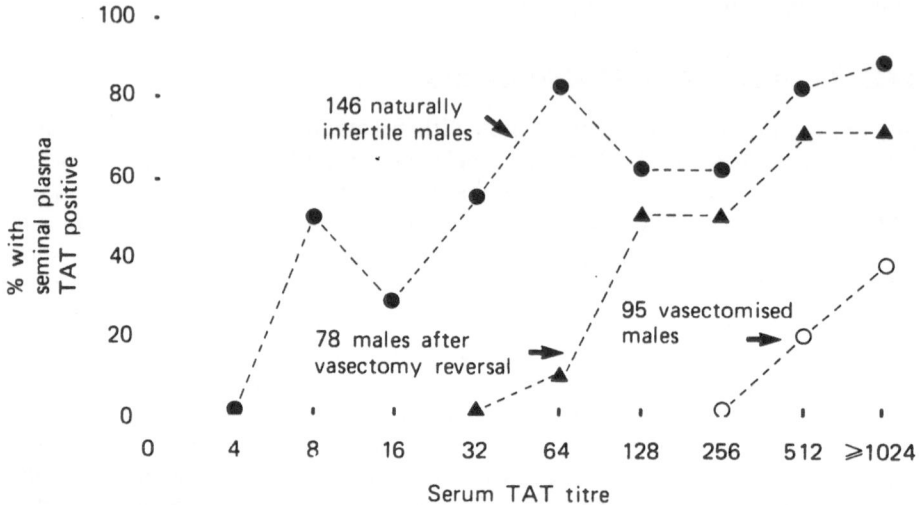

Figure 6.1 Proportion of patients with seminal plasma antisperm antibodies related to serum titre, comparing spontaneously infertile males with vasectomised men before and after reversal.

About one-third of subfertile men with antisperm antibodies have oligozoospermia (Rumke and Hellinga, 1959), but it is not clear whether the antibodies caused the low sperm count (Rumke, 1981). Certainly immune orchitis can be induced experimentally in animals (Waksman, 1959) and man (Mancini *et al.*, 1965). The main sites affected are the head of the epididymis, which becomes plugged with polymorphonuclear leucocytes, and in and around the rete testis, where mononuclear cells infiltrate the interstitium, although infiltration of the seminiferous tubules is uncommon. This is considered to be because the rete testis and epididymis are the weakest points in the blood–testis barrier (Brown and Glynn, 1969). Thus there may be a cell-mediated component of the antisperm antibody reaction in sub-fertile men resulting in partial blockage to sperm flow in the efferent passages, which could contribute to the infertility by producing oligozoospermia (see below).

ANTISPERM ANTIBODIES AND TESTICULAR OBSTRUCTION

After experimental vasoligation in animals, testicular lymph and regional lymph nodes consistently contain spermatozoa (Ball and Setchell, 1983), and spermatozoa have been found in a para-aortic lymph node one year after vasectomy in a man undergoing laparotomy (Ball *et al.*, 1982). It is, therefore, not surprising that antisperm antibodies develop in the serum of 60–80% of men following vasectomy (Hellema and Rumke, 1978; Rose and Lucas, 1979).

We measured antisperm antibodies in serum and seminal plasma in 130 males before and after vasectomy reversal, and the occurrence of pregnancy was analysed in those partners who were trying to produce a pregnancy. All patients were followed for at least one year. Sperm agglutinating antibodies were found in the serum of 79% of patients; seminal plasma antibodies were present in only 9.5% before reversal, and this rose to 29.5% afterwards (Parslow *et al.*, 1983). Overall, pregnancies occurred in the partners of 44.6% of those men who were trying to produce children. Production of pregnancy was significantly less likely when the pre-operative serum antisperm antibody titre was ≥ 512, but no decrease in fertility was seen with titres below this. Similar numbers of pregnancies were produced by patients with or without seminal plasma antibodies, in titres of up to 16. This is different from the findings in spontaneously infertile males (see above).

Further studies have shown that this distinction is probably due to the antibodies being of a different class. Most of the antibody produced after vasectomy is IgG, and some may transude from serum into the seminal plasma, whereas in spontaneously infertile males much of the seminal plasma antibody is IgA probably produced locally in the genital tract. It appears that the locally produced IgA exerts a more powerful adverse effect on fertility (Parslow *et al.*, 1985).

The spontaneously infertile male with azoospermia differs from the vasectomised male in a number of respects. If the block is congenital, many years will have elapsed since the antigenic stimulus first appeared, and since the induction of the immune response was gradual, a degree of tolerance may have occurred. With acquired, post-infective blocks on the other hand the obstruction followed an acute inflammatory disease of the genital system that may well have stimulated considerably more local antibody formation than the comparatively clean surgical procedure of vasectomy In 168 azoospermic males, we found that serum antisperm antibodies occurred approximately twice as often in the acquired as in the congenital groups. After surgical correction of azoospermia, production of pregnancy was significantly more likely in those patients who did not have such antibodies (by Fisher's exact test, $p < 0.05$), (Hendry *et al.*, 1985). It is thus possible that antisperm antibodies may have different and more potent effects in patients with acquired post inflammatory blocks than in men undergoing vasectomy reversal.

TREATMENT

Therapy for antisperm antibodies is demanding on the time of clinical and laboratory staff, and requires great patience and perseverance from the subfertile couple concerned. It can also produce serious side effects. It is therefore necessary to make quite sure before starting treatment (i) that the antisperm antibodies are really interfering with fertility, (ii) that the husband's sperm count is as good as possible, and (iii) that the wife has patent tubes and that the presence and timing of ovulation has been established. Close liaison between the staff looking after husband and wife are essential.

There are three possible lines of treatment, and none are completely satisfactory at present.

A. Antibiotics. Prostatitis has been noted in a high proportion (37%) of 43 men with antisperm antibodies in Sweden (Fjallbrant and Obrant, 1968). A significant decrease in antibody titre was observed following prolonged antibiotic treatment (for up to 3 years) in eight cases, with pregnancies in five of the wives (Fjallbrant and Nilsson, 1977).

B. Artificial insemination – sperm washing. Kremer *et al.* (1978c) have used intrauterine insemination to get beyond the barrier created by the cervical mucus, and obtained three pregnancies (including one abortion) in 15 women. We have treated 30 couples with production of only three pregnancies.

C. Steroids. Before giving steroids we check for a family history of diabetes or glycosuria, measure the fasting blood sugar, check liver function tests, and do a chest X-ray. Dyspepsia is fully investigated and treated prior to and during

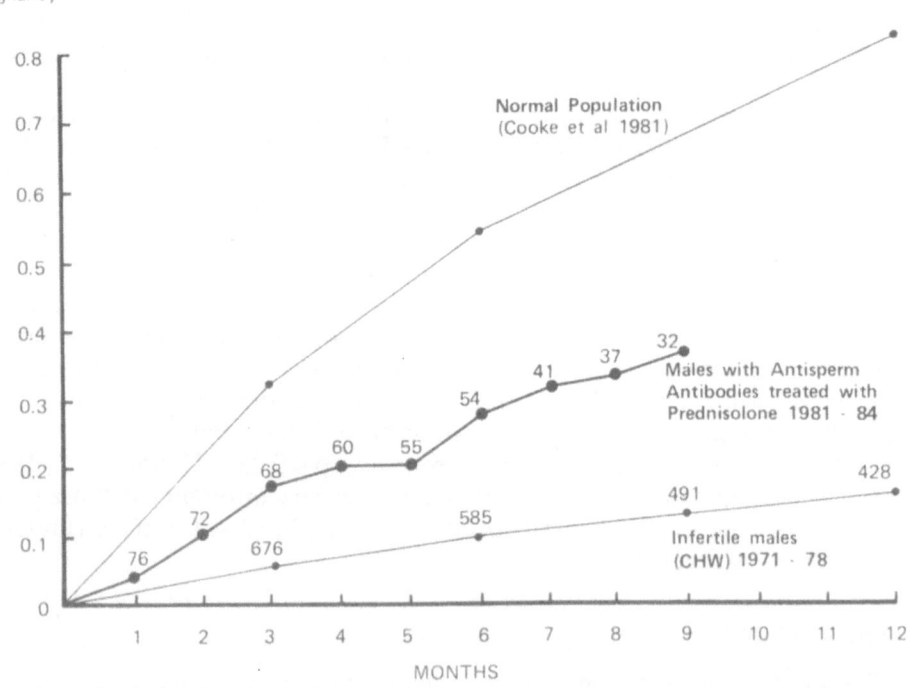

Figure 6.2 Pregnancies produced by subfertile males with antisperm antibodies during intermittent prednisolone therapy, compared to the normal population and an unselected group of infertile males (from Hendry *et al.*, 1986).

therapy. Patients are told of the risks involved, and advised to abstain from alcohol whilst on treatment.

1.   Cyclical prednisolone therapy. Seventy-six subfertile males with significant titres of antisperm antibodies have been treated with a new corticosteroid regimen, consisting of prednisolone 40 mg daily, rising to 80 mg daily if antibody titres did not fall, given from day 1 to day 10 of the partner's menstrual cycle followed by 5 mg in the morning of days 11 and 12, for up to 9 cycles. Twenty-five (33%) of the partners became pregnant during a treatment cycle, over twice the expected incidence without treatment (Figure 6.2). No serious complications occurred, although half of the patients had transient minor side effects. This regimen appears to be encouraging and suitable for further assessment in a prospective controlled trial (Hendry et al., 1986).

2.   Long term low dose prednisolone therapy. Two patients with azoospermia had empty epididymes with normal spermatogenesis and very high antisperm antibody titres (> 1024). Following treatment with prednisolone 15 mg daily for six months, the sperm count rose to 17 m/ml in one case and to 26 m/ml in the other, falling back to less than 1 m/ml when prednisolone was discontinued. Testicular biopsy in three of these cases showed focal mononuclear cell infiltration of seminiferous tubules, suggesting **immune orchitis** (Hendry, 1987).

The fertility of some, but certainly not all, men with antisperm antibodies can be improved with steroids. Continuous therapy could be preferable initially for patients with severe oligozoospermia and high titres of antibodies, since the sperm count may rise to normal. Cyclical treatment is probably better if the sperm count is normal, although care should be taken to synchronise treatment with the wife's cycle. Repeated checking of post-coital tests and antisperm antibody titres gives a useful indication of the degree of response shown by the patient. In suitable cases the two regimes can be combined, or linked with artificial insemination, with or without sperm washing, or in vitro fertilisation.

     D. Unilateral orchidectomy.   Seven cases have been seen where unilateral testicular obstruction was associated with very high anti-sperm antibody titres and severe oligozoospermia, which improved after removal of the obstructed testis with production of two pregnancies. So it seems that a **secondary** immune orchitis affect the contralateral testis in patients with unilateral obstruction, which may respond to orchidectomy, followed if necessary by corticosteroid therapy. The existence of such obstruction might be clinically unsuspected, yet clearly the diagnosis should be established in a subfertile male, since correction of the block or removal of the obstructed testis could lead to restoration of fertility (Hendry, 1986).

CONCLUSIONS

Antisperm antibodies can significantly impair fertility in the male, and yet they may not be suspected at all unless specific tests are done to detect them. Once their existence has been recognised, the quantity, distribution and class of antibody should be defined before deciding on their likely significance. Although no precipitating cause can be defined in most cases, the possibility of unilateral testicular obstruction should be suspected, and either corrected if possible, or consideration should be given to removal of the obstructed testis, to eliminate the stimulus to continuing antibody production. In selected cases, intermediate dose cyclical, or long term low dose prednisolone therapy can be given, first to improve semen quality and secondly to increase the likelihood of pregnancy in the spouse. If the pregnancy does not occur spontaneously there is good evidence from recent experience that *in vitro* fertilisation may be successful following prednisolone treatment of male antisperm antibodies, where failure of sperm egg fusion may have occurred apparently due to the antisperm anti-bodies before such treatment.

References

Ball, R.Y. and Setchell, B.P. (1983). The passage of spermatozoa to regional lymph nodes in testicular lymph following vasectomy in rams and boars. *J. Reprod. Fertil.*, **68**, 145–153

Ball, R.Y., Naylor, C.P.E. and Mitchinson, M.J. (1982). Spermatozoa in an abdominal lymph node after vasectomy in a man. *J. Reprod. Fertil.*, **66**, 715–16

Brown, P.C. and Clynn, L.E. (1969). The early lesson of experimental allergic architis in guinea pigs: an immunological correlation. *J. Pathol.*, **98**, 277–82

Fjallbrant, B. (1968). Interrelation between high levels of sperm antibodies, reduced penetration of cervical mucus by spermatozoa, and sterility in men. *Acta Obstetrica et Gynaecologica Scandinavica*, **47**, 102–17

Fjallbrant, B. and Obrant, O. (1968). Clinical and survival findings in men with sperm antibodies. *Acta Obstet. Gynaecol. Scand.*, **47**, 451–68

Fjallbrant, B. and Nilsson, S. (1977). Decrease of sperm antibody titre in males and conception after treatment of chronic prostatitis. *Int. J. Fertil.*, **22**, 255–6

Friberg, J. (1974). A simple and sensitive micro-method for demonstration of sperm agglutinating antibodies in serum from infertile men and women. *Acta Obstet. Gynaecol. Scand.*, Supplement, **36**, 21–29

Halim, A. and Antoniou, D. (1973). Autoantibodies to spermatozoa in relation to male infertility and vasectomy. *Br. J. Urol.*, **45**, 559-562

Hellema, H.W.J. and Rumke, P. (1978). Sperm autoantibodies as a consequence of vasectomy. I. Within one year post-operation. *Clin. Exp. Immunol.*, **31**, 18–29.

Hendry, W.F. (1986). The clinical significance of unilateral testicular obstruction in subfertile males. *Br. J. Urol.*, **58**, 709–14

Hendry, W.F. (1987). Surgery for testicular obstruction. In Hendry, W.F. (ed.) *Recent Advance in Urology Andrology* 4. pp. 313–38 (Edinburgh: Churchill Livingstone)

Hendry, W.F., Morgan, H. and Stedronska, J. (1977). The clinical significance of anti-sperm antibodies in male subfertility. *Br. J. Urol.*, **49**, 757–62

Hendry, W.F. Parslow, J.M. and Stedronska, J. (1983). Exploratory scrototomy in 168 azoospermic males. *Br. J. Urol.*, **55**, 785–91

Hendry, W.F., Treehuba, K., Hughes, L., Stedronska, J., Parslow, J.M., Wass, J.A.H. and Besser, G.M. (1986). Cyclic prednisolone therapy for male infertility associated with antibodies to spermatozoa. *Fertil. Steril.*, **45**, 249–54

Husted, S. (1975). Immobilising and cytotoxic sperm antibodies in serum and seminal plasma and their relation to other sperm antibodies. *Acta Pathol. Microbiol. Scand.*, **83**, 338–46

Jager, S., Kremer, J. and Van Slochternen–Draaisma, T. (1978). A simple method of screening for antisperm antibodies in human males. *Int. J. Fertil.*, **23**, 12–21

Kremer, J., Jager, S. and Van Slochteren–Draaisma, T. (1978a). The 'unexplained' poor postcoital test. *Int. J. Fertil.*, **23**, 277–81.

Kremer, J., Jager, S., Kuiken, J. and Van Slochteren–Draaisma, T. (1978b). Recent advances in diagnosis and treatment of infertility due to antisperm antibodies. In Cohen, J. and Hendry, W.F. (eds.) *Spermatozoa Antibodies and Infertility*. pp. 117–27 (Oxford: Blackwells)

Kremer, J., Jager, S. and Kuiken, J. (1978c). Treatment of infertility caused by anti-sperm antibodies. *Int. J. Fertil.*, **23**, 270–6

Macleod, J. (1951). Semen quality in 1000 men of known fertility and in 800 cases of infertile marriage. *Fertil. Steril.*, **2**, 115–39

Macleod, J. and Gold, R.Z. (1951). The male factor in fertility and infertility IV. Sperm morphology in fertile and infertile marrage. *Fertil. Steril.*, **2**, 394–414

Mancinic, R.E., Andrada, J.A., Sarceni, D., Bachmann, A.E., Lavieri, J.C. and Nemirovsky, M. (1965). Immunological and testicular response in men sensitised with human testicular homogenate. *J. Clin. Endocrinol. Metab.*, **25**, 859–75

Morgan, H., Stedronska, J., Hendry, W.F., Chamberlain, G.V.P. and Dewhurst, C.J. (1977). Sperm/cervical mucus crossed hostility testing and antisperm antibodies in the husband. *Lancet*, **1**, 1228–30

Parslow, J.M., Royle, M.G., Kingscott, M.M.B., Wallace, D.M.A. and Hendry, W.F. (1983). The effects of sperm antibodies on fertility after vasectomy reversal. *Am. J. Rep. Immunol.*, **3**, 28–31

Parslow, J.M., Poulton, T.A., Besser, G.M. and Hendry, W.F. (1985). The clinical relevance of classes of immunoglobulins on spermatozoa from infertile and vasectomised males. *Fertil. Steril.*, **43**, 621–7

Rose, N.R. and Lucas, P.L. (1979). Immunological consequences of vasectomy II Two-year summary of prospective study. In Lepow, I.H. and Crozier, R. (eds.) *Vasectomy: Immunologic and Pathophysiologic Effects in Animals and Man*. pp. 533–60 (New York: Academic Press)

Rose, N.R., Hjort, J., Rumke, P., Harper, M.J.K. and Vyazov, O. (1976). Techniques for detection of iso and auto antibodies to human spermatozoa. *Clin. Exp. Immunol.*, **23**, 175–99

Rumke, P. (1978). Autoantigenicity of spermatozoa. In Cohen, J. and Hendry, W.F. (eds.) *Spermatozoa, Antibodies and Infertility*. pp.67–79 (Oxford: Blackwells)

Rumke, P. (1981). Can oligozoospermia be induced by autoimmunity? In Frajese, G., Hafez, E.S.E., Conti, C. and Fabrini, A. (eds.) *Oligozoospermia: Recent Progress in Andrology*. pp. 185–97 (New York: Raven Press)

Rumke, P. and Hellinga, G. (1959). Autoantibodies against spermatozoa in sterile men. *Am. J. Clin. Pathol.*, **32**, 357–63

Rumke, P., Van Amstel, N., Messer, E.N. and Bezemer, P.D. (1974). Prognosis of fertility of men with sperm agglutinins in the serum. *Fertil. Steril.*, **25**, 393–8

Santomauro, A.G., Sciarra, J.J. and Varma, A.O. (1972). A clinical investigation of the role of semen analysis and post-coital test in the evaluation of male infertility. *Fertil. Steril.*, **23**, 245–51

Stedronska, J. and Hendry, W.F. (1983). The value of the mixed antiglobulin reaction (MAR test) as an addition to routine seminal analysis in the evaluation of the subfertile couple. *Am. J. Rep. Immunol.*, **3**, 89–91

Stedronska-Clarke, J., Clarke, D.A. and Hendry, W.F. (1987). Antisperm antibodies detected by ZER enzyme linked immunosorbent assay are not those detected by Tray Aggutination Test. *Am. J. Rep. Immunol. Microbiol.*, **13**, 76–7

Waksman, B.H. (1959). A histologic study of the auto allergic testis lesion in the guinea pig. *J. Exp. Med.*, **109**, 311–24

WHO Reference Bank for Reproductive Immunology (1977). Auto- and iso-antibodies to antigens of the human reproductive system I. Results of an international comparative study. *Clin. Exp. Immunol.*, **30**, 173–80

DISCUSSION

Question: What is the evidence that in the human male, spermatozoa pass into the lymph nodes?

Hendry: A number of spermatozoa were identified in the lymph nodes of a man with Hodgkin's disease who had a vasectomy one year previously. (Ball, Naylor and Mitchinson, 1982, *J. Reprod. Fertil.*, **66**, 715–716).

Question: What is the role of infection in the production of antisperm antibodies?

Hendry: In our laboratories (Shahmanesh, Stedronska and Hendry 1986, *Fertil. Steril.*, **46**, 308–311) we examined men for anti-sperm antibodies who were presenting at a Genito-Urinary Medicine Department for NSU. Only a few men with NSU developed antisperm antibodies. As with other autoimmune disease the genetic make up of the individual is important in determining whether an insult will result in immunisation.

Question: Why are some patients with a titre of less than 32 treated with 40 mg Prednisolone?

Hendry: In these cases, patients had seminal plasma antibodies and impaired penetration of cervical mucus. We would not treat these patients if no seminal plasma antibodies were present. Occasionally, some patients have higher titres of seminal plasma than serum antibodies.

Question: In the cases of infiltration of the testis by lymphocytes was the semen examined for the presence of lymphocytes?

Hendry: No. It would be an easy way of detecting such cases without the need for a testicular biopsy if lymphocytes in the semen were indicative of an infiltration into the testis.

Question: Has cyclosporin A been used in the treatment of antisperm antibodies?

Hendry: Yes. It has been successfully used. A recent reference is Bouloux *et al.* (1986) *Fertil. Steril.*, **46**, 81–85.

A point of medico-legal interest: All patients must be warned if treatment for a medical condition is potentially dangerous on the grounds that they may opt not to follow your recommendation or treatment.

7
PRINCIPLES AND GUIDELINES FOR ANTISPERM ANTIBODY SCREENING

J.H. Adeghe, C.L.R. Barratt and J. Cohen

INTRODUCTION

A. General

Testing for antisperm antibodies (ASA) is an important step in the investigation of subfertile couples. The mechanisms by which ASA impair fertility, and indeed the detailed treatment of cases, are dealt with in Chapter 6 by W.F. Hendry. This chapter aims at those clinics interested in choosing, and setting up, techniques for ASA-testing as part of their armamentarium.

B. Who and what to test?

Traditionally, tests on blood serum have been used to identify men with ASA. This has been criticised (Beer and Neaves, 1978; Bronson, Cooper and Rosenfeld, 1984), and it has been argued that only the ASA present locally in semen would be expected to have any clinical relevance. Indeed, it has become clear that there is a dichotomy between local and systemic immune response to sperm; ASA may be present in serum but not in semen, or *vice versa*. A complete assessment of spermatozoal autoimmunity would therefore need to include tests on three compartments – serum, seminal plasma, and the sperm surface.

Because ASA-based infertility is relatively uncommon, many clinics choose to test for antibodies only in men who show 'suspicious' features in the seminal fluid analysis (SFA) or in sperm–cervical mucus interaction test. One such feature is the presence of spontaneous autoagglutination in ejaculates. However, using this criterion would be insufficient, as half of the men with ASA problems do not have such agglutination. Moreover, it is sometimes impossible, even for the experienced technician, to tell true agglutination from 'aggregation' resulting from adventitious bacteria or dirty glassware. Another widespread belief is that hypomotility of sperm is pathognomonic of antisperm antibodies; however, objective confirmation is necessary. When we examined this experimentally, using Timed Exposure Photomicrography, we found no relationship between sperm movement kinetics and the presence of spermagglutinating or immobilizing antibodies in seminal plasma. A poor post-coital test, or 'shaking' found during in vitro sperm-penetration test, are also used as criteria for ASA testing, but these only indicate high levels of IgA antibodies in semen or cervical mucus; good mucus penetration can occur in the presence of IgG–ASA, (Parslow et al., 1985; Wang et al., 1985).

Because the so-called 'suspicious signs' may often be inconclusive (in either direction), the logical thing would be to test all the male partners of infertile couples, perhaps as part of routine SFA's.

THE LABORATORY TESTS

General principles

Techniques for detecting ASA in serum or semen are mostly based on one or more of the following principles:

1. Agglutination – results when multivalent antibodies cause adherence between spermatozoa by cross-linking them. Such agglutination may be detectable microscopically or macroscopically.

   The Gelatin Agglutination Test (GAT; also called Kibrick-method; Kibrick, Belding and Merrill, 1952) is an example of a macro-agglutination test.

   Micro-agglutination tests include: Slide agglutination test (SAT; Rumke and Hellinga, 1959) Modified slide agglutination test (MSAT; Francavilla et al., 1983) Tube–slide agglutination test (TSAT; also called Franklin–Dukes method; Franklin and Dukes, 1964a,b) Tray agglutination test (TAT; Friberg, 1974).

2. Complement-dependent immobilization cytotoxicity – results from binding of antibody molecules to sperm surface antigens, which activates complement resulting in disruption of sperm membranes. The ultimate effect on sperms can be detected microscopically as a loss of motility (immobilization) or cell permeability leading rapidly to death (cytotoxicity). Several methods have been used for measuring immobilizing or cytoxic activity. These include the methods of Fjallbrant (1969), Hamerlynck and Rumke (1968), Isojima, Li and Ashitaka (1968), Husted and Hjort (1975), and Hellema and Rumke (1978).

3. Reaction between antibody-coated sperm and antiglobulin conjugated with various biological, chemical or synthetic materials, such as:
   (a) Fluorescein: in immunofluorescent techniques (Hansen and Hjort, 1971; Hjort and Hansen, 1971).
   (b) Enzymes: in Enzyme-linked Immunosorbent Assay (ELISA; Zanchetta, Busola and Mastrogiacomo, 1982; Alexander and Bearwood, 1984; Wolff and Schill, 1985)
   (c) Radioactive materials: in radiolabelled-antiglobulin technique (Haas, Cines and Schreiber, 1980)

(d)   Red blood cells: in mixed antiglobulin reaction (MAR test; Coombs, 1962; Coombs, Rumke and Edwards, 1973; Jager, Kremer and Van Slochteren–Draaisma, 1978)

(e)   Polyacrylamide microspheres: in Immunobead Test (IBT; Bronson, Cooper and Rosenfeld, 1981; Clarke, Stojanoff and Cauchi, 1982).

(f)   Surfaces of wells in plastic trays: in 'Panning' (Hancock and Faruki, 1984)

B. Which test?

Detailed critical reviews and studies on various ASA tests have been provided by Shulman (1975), Beer and Neaves (1978), Jones (1980a,b), Menge (1980), and World Health Organization (WHO) sponsored multicentre studies (Rose *et al.*, 1976; Boettcher *et al.*, 1977; Bronson *et al.*, 1985). Based on such reports, Table 7.1 lists advantages and drawbacks of some tests, and so shows constraints on our choice of tests for clinical use. In making the decision as to which test to act upon, we direct your attention to the following:

1.   Antibodies present locally (especially on the sperm surface) are more immediately relevant to fertility status than those in the blood.

2.   It is not sufficient merely to demonstrate the presence of antibodies; their immunoglobin class and surface specificity are very important clinical indicators for aetiology and treatment.

3.   No one test is sufficient to provide all relevant information on a patient's autoimmunity to sperm; it usually requires a combination of tests, perhaps two (e.g. Immunobead test for sperm surface antibodies and TAT for spermagglutinating activity in seminal plasma and serum) performed on at least two occasions.

4.   Some tests are excluded by cost; simple and inexpensive techniques, not requiring elaborate equipment or too much of the technician's time, are better suited for use on a routine basis.

Table 7.1 Advantages/drawbacks of some antisperm antibody tests (See text for references)

Technique	Comments
1. Immunofluorescence (IF)	Tedious; very stringent controls and the utmost care in the laboratory are required; nevertheless results correlate poorly with clinical findings (Hendry et al., 1978).
2. Gelatin Agglutination Test (GAT)	Reproducible and specific; presence of agglutination is observed by the naked eye so microscope is not required. However, it requires relatively large volumes of semen; the part of each sperm involved in the agglutination cannot be read; sensitivity of H–H agglutination is low (Hellema and Rumke, 1976).
3. Tube–Slide Aggluttination Test (TSAT)	Detects mainly H–H agglutination; probably not useful for testing male sera where T–T agglutination is most common.
4. Tray Agglutination Test (TAT)	Sensitive for all types of agglutination; requires small volumes of reagents, so large number of samples can be tested simultaneously with one donor semen sample (and thawed control samples); type of agglutination can be observed directly but requires an inverted microscope (and some expertise in its use) which some labs do not have.
5. Modified Slide Agglutination Test (MSAT)	Utilizes all the technical advantages of TAT, and is done on glass slides, rather than in multiwell trays; therefore requires an ordinary microscope. Sensitivity similar to that of TAT.
6. Sperm Immobilization Test (SIT)	Less sensitive but more specific than agglutination tests; it is of no additional diagnostic benefit (no more than agglutination test). May be useful in monitoring response to treatment.
7. Mixed Antiglobulin Reaction (MAR)	Inexpensive and simple to use, IgG–MAR test is fairly sensitive, and correlates well with TAT on serum. IgA–MAR test is probably not as sensitive as its IgG counterpart. MAR test depends on presence of motile sperm in semen. Results are difficult to quantitate accurately.
8. Immunobead Test (IBT)	Simple, sensitive and specific. Allows determination of isotype and surface location of antibodies. Also depends on presence of motile sperm.
9. Enzyme Linked Immunosorbent Assay (ELISA)	Correlates poorly with other common tests; lacks standardization. Potentially useful.
10. 'Panning' Assay	Simple to use; allows testing of sperm with poor motility; clinical trial is not yet available.

C. Recommendations

We strongly recommend the Immunobead test or the IgG–MAR test for sperm surface antibodies, and the Tray agglutination test or Modified slide agglutination test for spermagglutinating antibodies in blood serum or seminal plasma.

Detailed 'cook-book' recipes of each of these techniques will not be given, as this is not intended to serve as a laboratory manual instead of the published method. We would rather emphasize the need for stringent quality control, and provide suggestions for achieving this.

1. *Immunobead Test (IBT).* Immunobead reagents are available commercially (Bio-Rad Labs) and consist of polyacrylamide microspheres coated covalently with Rabbit Antihuman immunoglobulins; each reagent category is reactive against one immunoglobulin class. Thus, Antihuman-IgA, -IgG, -IgM immunobeads are available. The technique is well described in Bronson, Cooper and Rosenfeld (1981), Clarke, Elliot and Smaila, (1985), and Adeghe, Cohen and Sawers (1986). Basically, it consists of mixing washed sperm with a suspension of immunobeads on a glass slide; this is left to incubate for 5–10 minutes at 37°C or at room temperature. Samples of each ejaculate are tested separately for each immunoglobulin class of antibodies. After the incubation period, at least 200 motile sperm are scored for (a) the proportion of sperm with beads sticking to them, expressed as a percentage (% sperm binding), and (b) the part of the sperm to which the beads are stuck. There is no general agreement as to what constitutes a positive test. A positive sperm binding of 10 is regarded as positive by Bronson, Cooper and Rosenfield (1981) and Adeghe, Cohen and Sawers (1986); 20 by Clarke *et al.* (1985); and 50 by Jennings, McGowan and Baker (1985). Due to this lack of uniformity in classifying results, each laboratory should establish its own level of non-specific binding by determing the mean % sperm binding in a group of men with a recent history of fertility (as defined later under 'Protocol for Quality Control').

   Immunobead test should also be used as an indirect test, to determine the presence and class of antibodies in serum or seminal plasma. In such tests, antibodies are passively transferred to donor sperm which are washed then incubated in the test medium; they are then washed again and tested with immunobeads.

2. *Mixed Antiglobulin Reaction (MAR Test).* This was first used to study antisperm antibodies by Coombs (1962), Jeffrey and Parish (1972), Coombs, Rumke and Edwards (1973). But the report of Jager, Kremer and Van Slochteren–Draaisma (1978) standardised the technique as a screening method for sperm surface IgG-antibodies. The usefulness of the test was subsequently confirmed by Hendry and Stedronska (1980). The test system involves mixing, on a microscope slide, of one drop each of fresh semen, sensitized Group O Rh +ve red blood cells (RBC's), and monospecific anti-human IgG. If spermatozoa carry IgG on their surface, then a mixed agglutination is observed, and motile sperm can be seen attaching to clumps of red blood cells.

   Agglutination of the RBC's constitutes an internal control for each test; failure of RBC agglutination invalidates the test. Coating of the RBC's with 'incomplete Anti-D IgG' is important for success of the test. This is anti-rhesus D serum, incubated briefly with papain to free Fab fragments which attach specifically to the Rhesus positive blood cells. It is a good idea to arrange with a nearby haematology department to assist in preparing the sensitized cells.

3.   *Tray Agglutination Test (TAT).* This was first used by Friberg (1974), and has since become established as the most sensitive test for serum/seminal plasma spermagglutinins (Linnet and Suonimen, 1982). In performing the test, serial two-fold dilutions of test samples are made, and 5 μl of each dilution is mixed with 1 μl of donor sperm, in the wells of a microtitre tray. Each drop of mixture is covered with a layer of paraffin-oil and incubated at room temperature (for 4 hours) or at 37°C (for 2 hours). Each is then examined microscopically for the presence, degree and type of agglutination (inverted microscopy is preferred, viewing through the flat Petri base rather than the paraffin-oil).

4.   *Modified Slide Agglutination Test (MSAT).* This was described by Francavilla *et al.* (1983) and is based on the same principle and technique as the TAT, except the MSAT is performed on microscope slides. Observation can therefore be done with ordinary microscopes (not an inverted microscope – which most semenology labs do not have). This system provides for easier microscopy (and even better optics!) than in TAT. We have found the MSAT to have similar sensitivity to the TAT.

Protocol for quality control

In our opinion, establishing and maintaining stringent quality control measures for these tests is crucial. The following measures are recommended.

A.   Laboratories should collect and test 'suspect samples' (e.g. serum from vasectomized men; seminal plasma and sperm from men who have had vasectomy-reversal). Positive samples should then be pooled, refrozen in hundreds of small aliquants and stored. Normal samples should be collected from men with a recent history of fertility (less than 1 year; preferably husbands of pregnant wives or donors in a donor insemination programme) and frozen in small aliquants. The laboratory would therefore have generated its own controls; each patient test should be accompanied by positive and negative controls. The laboratory can then set its own standards and monitor its own consistency.

B.   Fresh donor semen, when required for a test, should be of the highest quality. Samples with many round cells, debris, poor sperm motility or low sperm count should never be used.

C.   Every new batch of commercially available products should first be tested for effectiveness. For example, Immunobeads should be tested against known ASA-positive and ASA-negative sperm sample (your standard aliquants) before testing patients' samples.

D.   High standards of cleanliness of laboratory glasswares and plasticware must be maintained, especially with glass slides and coverslips, because many bacterial antigens (pyrogens) produce false positives.

References

Adeghe, A.J.H., Cohen, J. and Sawers, R.S. (1986). Relationship between local and systemic autoantibodies to sperm, and evaluation of immunobead test for sperm surface antibodies. *Acta Eur. Fertil.*, **17**, 99–105

Alexander, N.J. and Bearwood, D. (1984). An immunosorption assay for antibodies to spermatozoa in comparison with agglutination and immobilization tests. *Fertil.Steril.*, **41**, 270–6

Beer, A.E. and Neaves, W.B. (1978). Antigenic status of semen from the viewpoints of the female and male. *Fertil. Steril.*, **29**, 3–22

Boettcher, B., Hjort, T., Rumke, P.L., Shulman, S. and Vyavoz, O. (1977). Auto- and iso-antibodies of the human reproductive system. I. Results of an international comparative study. *Clin. Exp. Immunol.*, **30**, 173–80

Bronson, R., Cooper, G., Hjort, T., Ing, R., Jones, W.R., Wang, S.X., Mathur, S., Williamson, H.O., Rust, P.F., Fudenberg, H.H., Mettler, L., Czuppon, A.B. and Sudo, N. (1985). Antisperm antibodies detected by agglutination, immobilization, microcytotoxicity and immunobead binding assays. *J. Reprod. Immunol.*, **8**, 279–99

Bronson, R., Copper, G. and Rosenfeld, D. (1981). Ability of antibody-bound human sperm to penetrate zona-free hamster ova in vitro. *Fertil. Steril.*, **36**, 778–83

Bronson, R., Cooper, G. and Rosenfeld, D. (1984). Sperm antibodies: their role in infertility. *Fertil. Steril.*, **42**, 171–83

Clarke, G.N., Elliot, P.J. and Smaila, C. (1985). Detection of sperm antibodies in semen using the immunobead test: a survey of 813 consecutive patients. *Am. J. Reprod. Immunol.*, **7**, 118–23

Clarke, G.N., Stojanoff, A. and Cauchi, M.N. (1982). Immunologlobulin class of sperm-bound antibodies in semen. In Bratanov, K. (ed.) *Immunology of Reproduction.* pp 482–5. (Sofia: Bulgarian Academy of Science Press)

Coombs, R.R.A. (1962). Mixed agglutination reactions in relation to spermatozoa. In *Proceedings of a Conference on Immuno-reproduction.* pp. 127–32. (New York: The Population Council)

Coombs, R.R.A., Rumke, P. and Edwards, R.G. (1973). Immunoglobulin classes reactive with spermatozoa in the serum and seminal plasma of vasectomized and infertile men. In Bratanov, K., Edwards, R.G., Vulchanov, V.H., Dikov, V. and Somlev, B. (eds.) pp. 354–9. (Sofia: Bulgarian Academy of Science Press)

Fjallbrant, B. (1969). Studies on sera from men with sperm antibodies. *Acta Obstet. Gynecol. Scand.*, **48**, 131–46

Francavilla, F., Catignani, P., Romano, R., Santucci, R., Francavilla, S and Santiemma, V. (1983). Modification of the slide agglutination test for the detection of sperm-agglutins. *Andrologia*, **15**, 699–704

Franklin, R.R. and Dukes, C.D. (1964a). Antispermatozoal antibody and unexplained infertility. *Am. J. Obstet. Gynecol.*, **89**, 6–9

Franklin, R.R. and Dukes, C.D. (1964b). Further studies on sperm agglutinating antibody and unexplained infertility. *J. Am. Med. Assoc.*, **190**, 682–3

Friberg, J. (1974). A simple and sensitive micro-method for demonstration of sperm agglutinating activity in serum from infertile men and women. *Acta Obstet. Gynaecol. Scand.* Suppl., **36**, 21–29

Haas, G.G., Cines, D.B. and Schreiber, A.D. (1980). Immunologic infertility: Identification of patients with antisperm antibody. *N. Engl. J. Med.*, **303**, 722–7

Hamerlynck, J. and Rumke, P. (1968). A test for the detection of cytotoxic antibodies in men. *J. Reprod. Fertil.*, **17**, 191–4

Hancock, R.T.J. and Faruki, S. (1984). Detection of antibody-coated sperm by 'panning' procedures. *J. Immunol. Meth.*, **66**, 149–59

Hansen, K.B. and Hjort, T. (1971). Immunofluorescent studies on human spermatozoa. II Characterization of spermatozoal antigens and their occurrence in spermatozoa from male partners of infertile couples. *Clin. Exp. Immunol.*, **9**, 21–31

Hellema, H.W.T. and Rumke, P. (1976). Comparison of the tray agglutination technique with the gelatin agglutination technique for the detection of sperm agglutinating activity in human sera. *Fertil. Steril.*, **27**, 284–92

Hellema, H.W.J. and Rumke, P. (1978). The micro-sperm immobilization test: the use of only motile spermatozoa and studies of complement. *Clin. Exp. Immunol.*, **31**, 1–11

Hendry, W.F., Morgan, H. Stedronska, J., Scammell, G. and Chamberlain, G.V.P. (1978). The clinical significance of antisperm antibodies in male subfertility: cross hostility testing and prednisolone treatment. In Cohen, J. and Hendry, W. F. (eds.) *Spermatozoa, Antibodies and Infertility.* pp. 129–38. (Oxford: Blackwell Scientific Publications)

Hendry, W.F. and Stedronska, J. (1980). Mixed erythrocyte-spermatozoa antiglobulin reaction (MAR test) for the detection of antibodies against spermatozoa in infertile males. *J. Obstet. Gynecol.*, **1**, 59–62

Hjort, T. and Hansen, K.B. (1971). Immunofluorescent studies on human spermatozoa. I. The detection of different spermatozoal antibodies and their occurrence in normal and infertile women. *Clin. Exp. Immunol.*, **8**, 9–23

Husted, S. and Hjort, T. (1975). Microtechnique for simultaneous determination of immobilizing and cytotoxic sperm antibodies. *Clin. Exp. Immunol.*, **22**, 256–64

Isojima, S., Li, T.S. and Ashitaka, Y. (1968). Immunologic analysis of sperm immobilizing factor found in sera of women with unexplained sterility. *Am. J. Obstet. Gynecol.*, **101**, 677–83

Jager, S., Kremer, J. and Van Slochteren Draaisma, T. (1978). A simple method of screening for antisperm antibodies in the human male. *Int. J. Fertil.*, **23**, 12–21

Jeffrey, W. and Parish, W.E. (1972). Allergic infertility: laboratory techniques to detect antispermatozoal antibodies. *Clin. Allergy*, **2**, 261–79

Jennings, M.G., McGowan, M.P. and Baker, H.W.G. (1985). Immunoglobulins on human sperm: Validation of a screening test for sperm autoimmunity. *Clin. Reprod. Fertil.*, **3**, 335–42

Jones, W.R. (1980a). Immunological factors in male and female infertility. In Hears, J.P. (ed.) *Immunological Aspects of Reproduction and Fertility Control.* pp. 105–40. (Lancaster: MTP Press)

Jones, W.R. (1980b). Immunologic infertility: fact or fiction? *Fertil. Steril.*, **33**, 577–86

Kibrick, S., Belding, D.L. and Merrill, B. (1952). Methods for detection of antibodies against mammalian spermatozoa. II. A gelatin agglutination test. *Fertil. Steril.*, 3, 430–8

Linnet, L., Suonimen, J.J.O. (1982). A comparison of eight techniques for the evaluation of the auto–immune response to spermatozoa after vasectomy. *J. Reprod. Immunol.*, 4, 133–44

Menge, A.C. (1980). Clinical immunologic infertility: diagnostic measures, incidence of antisperm antibodies, fertility and mechanisms. In Dhindsa, D.S., Schumacher, G.F.B. (eds.) *Immunological Aspects of Infertility and Fertility Regulation.* pp. 205–24. (New York: Elsevier North Holland)

Parslow, J.M., Poulton, T.A., Besser, G.M. and Hendry, W.F. (1985). The clinical relevance of classes of immunoglobulins on spermatozoa from infertile men and vasovasostomized males. *Fertil. Steril.*, 43, 621–7

Rose, N.R., Hjort, T., Rumke, P., Shulman, S. and Vyazov, O.E. (1976). Techniques for detection of iso- and auto-antibodies to human spermatozoa. *Clin. Exp. Immunol.*, 23, 175–99

Rumke, P.L. and Hellinga, G. (1959). Autoantibodies against spermatozoa in sterile men. *Am. J. Clin. Pathol.*, 32, 357–63

Shulman, S. (1975). *Reproduction and Antibody Response.* (Cleveland: CRC Press)

Wang, C., Baker, H.W.G., Jennings, M.G., Burger, H.G. and Lutjen, P.L. (1985). Interaction between human cervical mucus and sperm surface antibodies. *Fertil. Steril.*, 44, 484–7

Wolff, H. and Schill, W.B. (1985). A modified enzyme linked immunosorbent assay for detection of antisperm antibodies. *Andrologia*, 17, 426–9

Zanchetta, R., Busolo, F., Mastrogiacomo, I. (1982). The enzyme-linked immunosorbent assay for detection of the antispermatozoal antibodies. *Fertil. Steril.*, 38, 730–4

8
HORMONAL INFLUENCES IN MALE INFERTILITY

F.H. Comhaire

INTRODUCTION

One of the major problems in evaluating the effect of treatment of male infertility is the fact that usually the male partner is not infertile, but subfertile, which means that his fertilizing potential is decreased rather than absent. Hence, spontaneous conceptions do occur. In order to prove a treatment to be effective, the pregnancy rate observed during treatment should significantly exceed the treatment-independent pregnancy rate. Therefore, it is important to study this 'spontaneous' pregnancy rate, before embarking on the discussion of possible treatments.

UNDERSTANDING SPONTANEOUS CONCEPTION RATES AND THEIR RELATION WITH DIFFERENT DEGREES OF SUBFERTILITY

In a first model we imagine a population of 100 couples all having an identical degree of fertility with 15% probability of conception per cycle. This value is close to the fertility of a normal, fertile population (Vessey *et al.*, 1978; Leridon, 1980). If all these couples try to achieve pregnancy starting at time zero, 15 (15% of 100) will be successful in the first cycle. Of the remaining 85 couples, 13 (15% of 85) will achieve a pregnancy in the second cycle, 11 (15% of 72) in the third cycle, etc. (Figure 8.1). After 12 cycles of exposure, 86 couples will have achieved success, whereas the remaining 14 couples will be considered infertile in agreement with the WHO working definition (World Health Organization, 1984). For each duration of exposure, the percentage of infertile couples can be calculated from formula I (Leridon, 1980) (Table 8.1). In the previous example the percentage of infertile couples will equal $(1 - 0.15)^{12}$ x 100 = 14% after 12 cycles, and $(1 - 0.15)^{24}$ x 100 = 2% after 24 cycles.

In the second model, we imagine a population of 100 couples with a reduced fertility and probability of conception of only 5% per cycle (Figure 8.2). If calculations are performed as above it will be found that $(1 - 0.05)12$ x 100 = 54% of the couples will remain infertile after 12 cycles, and $(1 - 0.05)^{24}$ x 100 + 29% after 24 cycles.

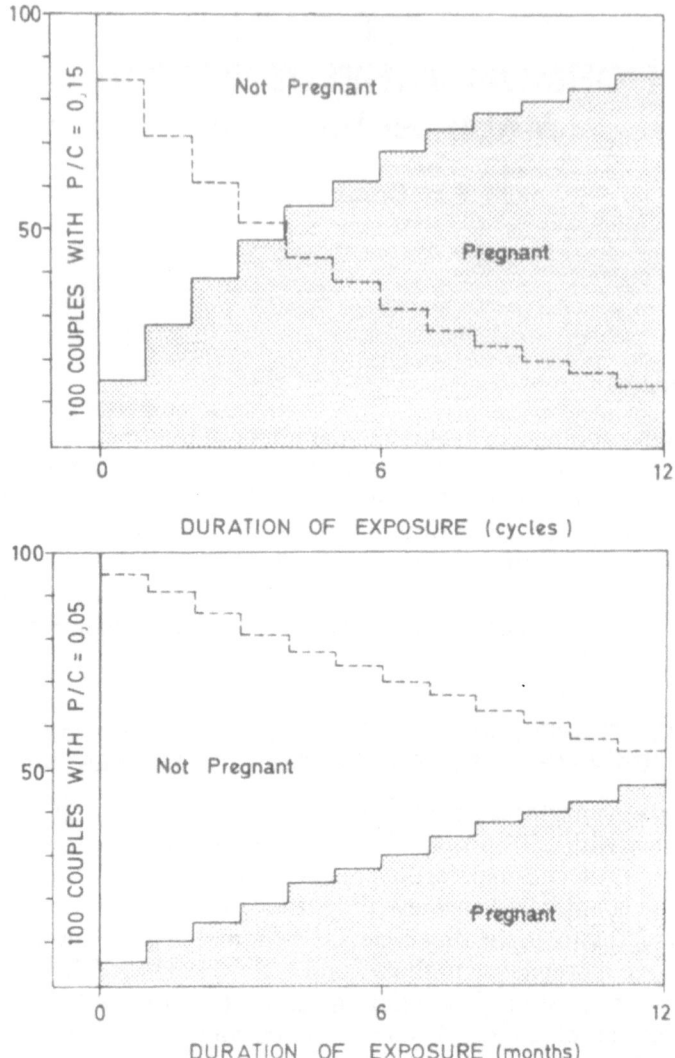

Figure 8.1

If all couples belonging to these two model populations and who have not achieved a pregnancy come to consultation after 12 cycles (1 year) of exposure, then there will be about four couples belonging to the group with low fertility for each couple belonging to the group with normal fertility (54 : 14 = 3.9) (Figure 8.3). If the infertile couples consult after 24 cycles (±2 years) of unsuccessful trial, the make-up of the population will differ with almost 15 couples belonging to the low-fertility group for each couple of the group with normal fertility (29 : 2 = 14.5).

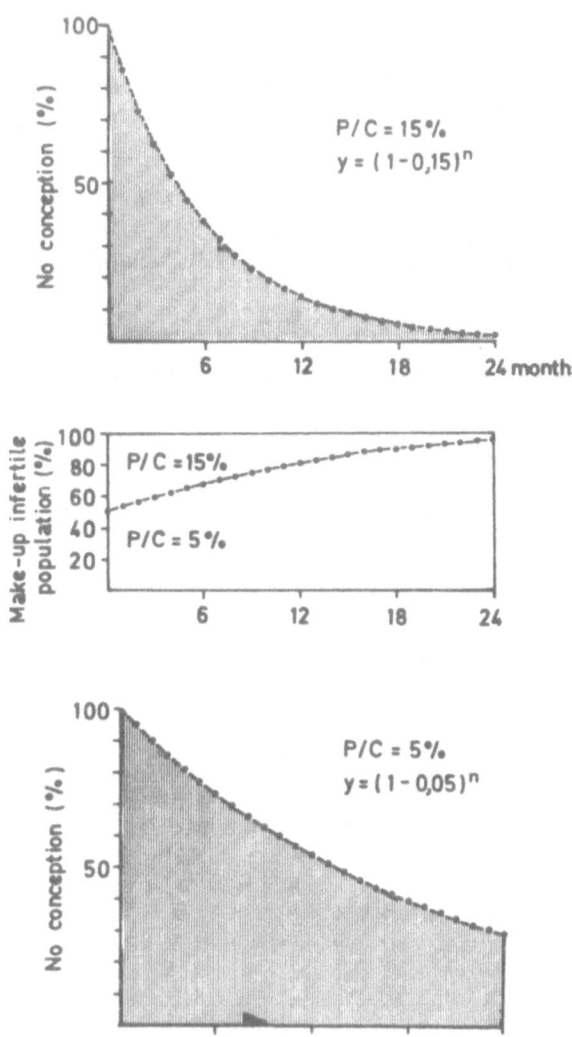

Figure 8.2

Table 8.1

Formula I

Proportion of infertile respectively fertile couples (in %) related to the conception rate per cycle (P/C, in %) and duration of exposure (n; number of cycles of trial to conceive).

infertile couples $= (1 - P/C)^n \times 100$
fertile couples $= [(1 - (1 - P/C)]^n \times 100$

Formula II

Probability of conception per cycle (P/C in %) related to the duration of infertility (x in months) in couples consulting for infertility
$$P/C = 4 \times 0.97^x$$

Formula III

Probability of conception per cycle (P/C in %) related to duration of infertility (x in months), type of infertility (a), severity of male factor (bm) and of female pathology (bf).

$$P/C = 4 \times 0.97^x \times (a) \times (bm) \times (bf)$$

Values for correction factors (a), (bm) and (bf) (calculated from Collins *et al.*, 1983, and Rousseau *et al.*, 1983)

(a)	primary infertility	=	0.9
	secondary infertility	=	1.35
(bm)	normal male	=	1.25
	moderate oligozoospermia (2 – 19.9 mill/m)	=	0.8
	severe oligozoospermia (0.1 – 1.9 mill/ml)	=	0.4
	azoospermia	=	0.08
(bf)	normal female age		
	20 – 30 y	=	1.25
	31 – 40 y	=	0.75
	40 y	=	0.50
	Type of pathology		
	– ovulatory disturbance	=	1.2
	– cervical factor	=	0.8
	– endometriosis	=	0.6
	– minor tubal pathology	=	0.6
	– bilateral tubal occlusion (diagnosed on HSG)	=	0.3

In analogy with the previous examples it is possible to calculate the composition of the infertile population in relation to the duration of infertility, when the original population consists of couples with a greatly variable probability of conception between 0 and 15% per cycle (Figure 8.4). If the previous reasoning is correct, the frequency of spontaneous pregnancies should decrease when the duration of infertility becomes longer, since the infertile population consists of an increasing proportion of couples with low probability of conception (Figure 8.4). Hence, the mean probability of conception for the entire population will decrease with time in spite of a constant probability of conception in each individual couple.

Data published on treatment-independent pregnancies in couples consulting for infertility are available on 4059 couples (Collins et al., 1983; Rousseau *et al.*, 1983; Hargreave and Nillson, 1984; Wood *et al.*, 1984) of which 1360

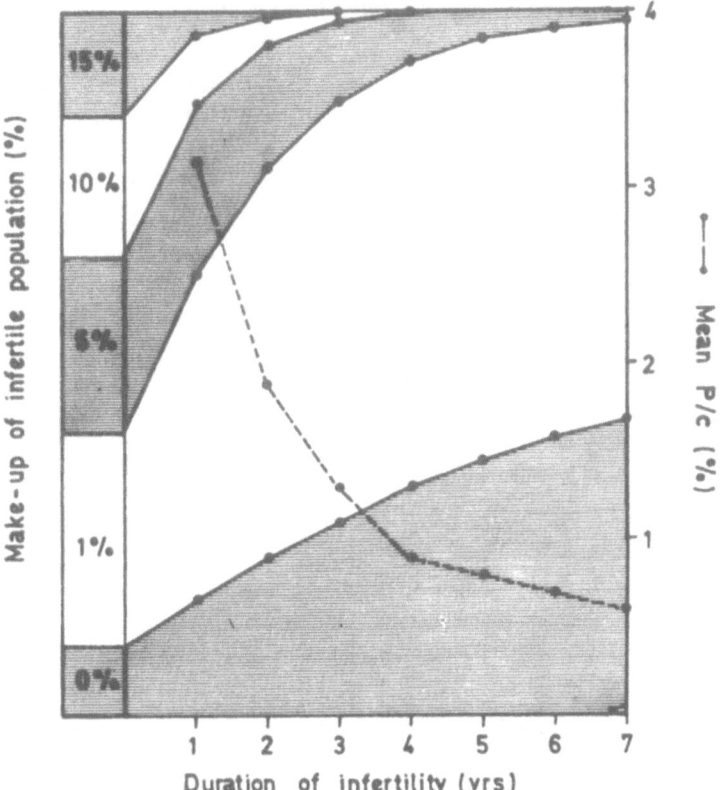

Figure 8.3

(33%) achieved pregnancy. Furthermore, data on spontaneous pregnancies have been analysed in a large population of 8350 couples investigated using a standardized protocol (World Health Organization, 1984) and of whom 753 (9%) achieved pregnancy during the work-up of their infertility problem. It appears that during the first 4 or 5 years of infertility, the relation between the frequency of spontaneous pregnancies and the duration of infertility is exponential. The line fitting the observed relation is described by a single logarithmic formula (formula II, Table 8.1) in which the duration of infertility has an exponential position.

Factors other than the duration of infertility may also influence the frequency of spontaneous pregnancies in couples consulting for infertility; the following seem to be of major importance (Collins *et al.*, 1983; Hargreave and Nillson, 1984; Wood *et al.*, 1984):

(a)   whether or not the couple has achieved a pregnancy previously (secondary versus primary infertility).

(bm) the degree of impairment of semen quality.

85

(bf)   age, type and severity of pathology of the female.

It appears that the type of pathology causing abnormal semen does not influence the male factor, which is determined only by the semen quality.

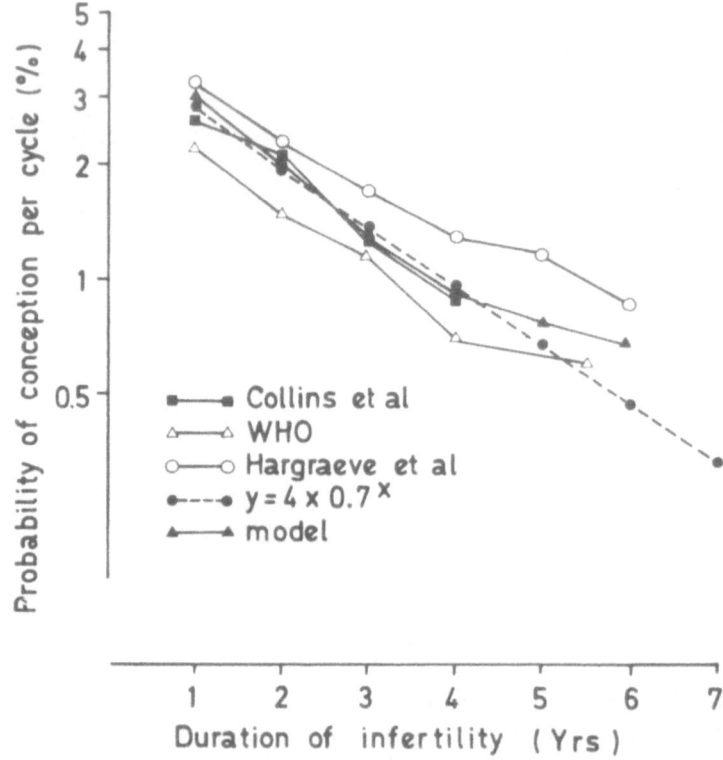

Figure 8.4

STUDY OF THE EFFECT OF TREATMENT ON INFERTILITY

Treatments of unproven value

Treatment of men with idiopathic testicular failure has been performed with all kinds of medications. Since controlled studies are lacking for the majority of these, their value should be considered unproven. Examples of such hormonal treatments of unproven value are:

–   High dose testosterone treatment using the Hellers' rebound method (Heller *et al.*, 1950).

- LHRH and its analogues, such as buserilin (Schwarzstein and Aparicio, 1982).

- Bromocriptine (Hovatta *et al.*, 1979; Masala *et al.*, 1979).

- Gonadotropins, either hCG, or hMG, or both combined (Sherins, 1974; Winters and Troen, 1982).

Treatments with doubtful effectiveness

Other treatments were reported to be successful in initial studies, but their benefit was not confirmed by other authors. Kallikrein stands as an example of these. Schill (1979) found oral kallikrein treatment to significantly improve sperm count and motility in a double-blind study. However, the duration of treatment was short (only 6 weeks) and the observed significance may be due rather to the fact that the placebo controls did not improve their semen quality, in contradistinction to what occurs usually.

In order to study the effect of any treatment, this should be given during at least 3 months, and preferably 6 months. Recently, oral kallikrein treatment of 3 months duration was found to be ineffective on the *in vitro* behaviour of spermatozoa tested by their capacity to migrate in buffer (Comhaire and Vermeulen, 1983) or in cervical mucus (Batterink *et al.*, 1983) or to fuse with zona free hamster ova (Comhaire and Vermeulen, 1983). These findings cast doubt on the effectiveness of oral kallikrein.

Treatments with presumed favourable effect

Until now, only two modes of hormonal treatment seem to stand the test of serious prospective studies, being the antioestrogens and mesterolone.

Mesterolone has been evaluated in a double-blind multicentre study by the World Health Organization (WHO, in preparation). Preliminary results suggest that a high dose treatment regimen of 150 mg/day doubles the pregnancy rate of patients with idiopathic infertility and oligozoospermia. However, the difference between treated patients and placebo controls is not significant and the study is continued by the recruitment of more cases.

Considering the fact that the effect of mesterolone is probably mediated through increased concentration of 5α-dihydrotestosterone, it seems sensible to undertake trials on the possible beneficial effect of testosterone undecanoate on objective sperm characteristics. Double blind investigations with high dose testosterone undecanoate (240 mg per day) are, in fact, being undertaken at the moment.

The antioestrogens clomiphene citrate (Ronnberg, 1980) and tamoxifen (Comhaire, 1976) have been reported to improve both semen quality and fertility in men with idiopathic infertility and oligozoospermia, as well as in patients remaining infertile after treatment of varicocele or male accessory gland infection. Clomiphene citrate is a racemic mixture and has a significant intrinsic

87

oestrogenic activity which may directly impair spermatogenesis (Schellen, 1982). Tamoxifen displays virtually no such oestrogenic activity and may be more suitable for treatment of the male (Comhaire, 1976).

Both drugs stimulate the pituitary gonadal axis by inhibiting the feed-back at the hypothalamic level, where testosterone is aromatized into oestradiol. This results in an enhanced secretion of LH and FSH and an increased production of 3 and 6 months of treatment in about 75% of patients (Vermeulen and Comhaire, 1978). All studies presently available report tamoxifen to improve fertility with overall pregnancy rate between 30 and 40% within one year; this is better than the pregnancy rate with placebo or with kallikrein treatment, being around 10–15% per year. Though a multicentre double-blind prospective study on tamoxifen treatment is still lacking, available data from randomized studies suggest this drug to be effective.

CONCLUSIONS

The evaluation of treatment of male infertility is extremely difficult and needs a major effort to be accomplished. Data presently available suggest that treatment with high dose mesterolone (150 mg/day) or with tamoxifen (20 mg/day) might improve fertility of patients with idiopathic infertility and moderate oligozoospermia, as well as in patients with persistent oligozoospermia after treatment for varicocele or male accessory gland infection. Simultaneous treatment of the female partner to optimalize her fertility may be helpful in increasing the success rate (Silber, 1983).

References

Batterink, G.J., Kremer, J. and Jager, S. (1983). The effect of oral kallikrein treatment on sperm motility in asthenozoospermia. *Int. J. Androl.*, **6**, 173–9

Collins, J.A., Wrixon, W., Janes, J.B. and Wilson, E.J. (1983). Treatment-independent pregnancy among infertile couples. *N. Engl. J. Med.*, **309**, 1201–6

Comhaire, F. (1976). Treatment of oligospermia with Tamoxifen. *Int. J. Fertil.*, **21**, 232–8

Comhaire, F. and Vermeulen, L. (1983). Effect of high dose oral Kallikrein treatment in men with idiopathic subfertility: evaluation by means of *in vitro* penetration test of zona free hamster ova. *Int. J. Androl.*, **6**, 168–72

Hargreave, T.B. and Nillson, S. (1984). Seminology. In Hargreave, T.B. (ed.) *Infertility.* pp. 56–74. (Berlin, Heidelberg, New York: Springer Verlag)

Heller, C.G., Nelson, W.O., Hill, I.B. *et al.* (1950). Improvement in spermatogenesis following depression of the human testis with testosterone. *Fertil. Steril.*, **1**, 415–22

Hovatta, O., Koskimies, A.I., Ranta, T. *et al.* (1979). Bromocriptine treatment of oligospermia: a double blind study. *Clin. Endocrinol.*, **11**, 377–82

Leridon, H. (1980). The efficacy of natural insemination: a comparative standard for AID. In David, G. and Price, W.S. (eds.) *Human Artificial Insemination and Semen Preservation.* pp. 191–6. (New York, London: Plenum Press)

Masala, A., Delitala, G., Algna, S. *et al.* (1979). Effects of long-term treatment with metergoline in patients with idiopathic oligospermia. *Clin. Endocrinol.*, 11, 349–52

Ronnberg, L. (1980). The effect of Clomiphene citrate on different sperm parameters and serum hormone levels in preselected infertile men: a controlled double-blind cross-over study. *Int. J. Androl.*, 3, 479–86

Rousseau, S., Lord, J., Lepage, Y. and Van Campenhout, J. (1983). The expectancy of pregnancy of 'normal' infertile couples. *Fertil. Steril.*, 6, 768–72

Schellen, A.M.C.M. (1982). Clomiphene citrate in the treatment of male infertility. In Bain, J., Schill, W.B. and Schwarzstein, L. (eds.) *Treatment of male infertility.* pp. 33–44. (Berlin, Heidelberg, New York: Springer Verlag).

Schill, W.B. (1979). Treatment of idiopathic oligozoospermia by Kallikrein: results of a double-blind study. *Arch. Androl.*, 2, 163–79

Schwarzstein, L. and Aparicio, N. (1982). LHRH and its analogs in the treatment of idiopathic normogonadotropic oligozoospermia. In Bain, J., Schill, W.B. and Schwarzstein, L. (eds.) *Treatment of Male Infertility.* pp. 57–69. (Berlin, Heidelberg, New York: Springer Verlag)

Sherins, R.J. (1974). Clinical aspects of treatment of male infertility with gonadotropins: testicular response of some men given hCG with and without Pergonal. In Mancini, R.E. and Martini, L (eds.) *Male Fertility and Sterility*, pp. 545–65. (London: Academic Press)

Silber, S.J. (1983). The use of Clomid for oligospermia: a controlled study; relationship to simultaneous treatment of the wife. *J. Androl.*, 4, 31 (abstract)

Vermeulen, A. and Comhaire, F. (1978). Hormonal effects of an anti-oestrogen. Tamoxifen in normal and oligospermic men. *Fertil. Steril.*, 29, 320–7

Vessey, M.P., Wright, N.H., McPherson, K. and Wiggins, P. (1978). Fertility after stopping different methods of contraception. *Br. Med. J.*, 1, 265–367

Winters, S.J. and Troen, P. (1982). Gonadotropin therapy in male infertility. In Bain, J., Schill, W.B. and Schwarzstein, L. (eds.) *Treatment of Male Infertility.* pp. 85–101. (Berlin, Heidelberg, New York: Springer Verlag)

Wood, C., Baker, G. and Trounson, A. (1984). Current status and future prospects. In Wood, C. and Trounson, A. (eds.) *Clinical In Vitro Fertilization.* pp. 11–26. (Berlin, Heidelberg, New York, Tokyo: Springer Verlag)

World Health Organization (1984). Workshop on the standardized investigation of the infertile couple. Moderator P. Rowe, Coordinator M. Darling. In Harrison, R.F., Bonnar, J. and Thompson, W. (eds.). *Proceedings of the 11th World Congress on Fertility and Sterility.* pp. 427–31. (Lancaster: MTP)

World Health Organization. (1987). Multicenter Study 78929: *Evaluation of Meterolone in the treatment of subfertile male.* (in preparation)

9
DIAGNOSIS AND DETECTION OF MALE ACCESSORY GLAND INFECTION

C.L.R. Barratt, T.C. Li and E.F. Monteiro

INTRODUCTION

During the conference there was concern over the conflicting data regarding the role of infection in male infertility. Although the diagnosis and management of male accessory gland infection (MAGI) is often difficult, costly and time consuming, the consensus of opinion was that only when its accurate detection was achieved and aetiological agent isolated could the role of this condition on male infertility be delineated.

The following chapter outlines the WHO diagnosis for MAGI (Comhaire et al., 1986). Its purpose is to outline the diagnosis and detection of MAGI but not discuss treatment or the effects of various infections on fertility. Those interested should refer to the following review articles (Keith et al., 1985a, 1985b; Fair & Sharer, 1986).

DEFINITION

MAGI includes inflammation of the prostate, epididymis and/or seminal vesicles (Comhaire et al., 1980). This may be associated with urethritis or urinary tract infection.

DIAGNOSTIC CRITERIA FOR MAGI

A. History and physical signs

1.   History – recurrent urinary tract infection and/or urethritis

2.   Physical signs – prostatitis and/or seminal vesiculitis and/or epididymitis and/or thickened vas deferens

B. Prostatic fluid signs

1.   Expressed prostatic secretion (EPS) >40 white blood cells per high powered field (WBC/HPF, HPF = x 400)

2.   Urinary sediment after prostatic massage > 15 WBC/HPF

3.   Positive bacterial culture in either EPS or post prostatic massage urine (Meares and Stamey, 1972).

C. Seminal signs

1.   Semen culture of 1 x 10^3 pathogenic bacteria/ml, or 1 x 10^4 non-pathogenic bacteria/ml (Comhaire et al., 1980).

2.   Semen containing more than 1 x 10^6 WBC/ml.

3.   Physical or biochemical abnormality of the seminal fluid i.e. low concentration of fructose, low activity of acid phosphatase, abnormal seminal pH, increased viscosity after liquifaction or the presence of mucus threads.
       Any of the above abnormalities may occur in isolation. The diagnosis of MAGI should therefore be based on a combination of signs and symptoms as follows:
       A history or physical sign with a prostatic fluid sign; or a history or physical sign with seminal sign; or a prostatic fluid sign with a seminal sign; or at least two seminal signs in each sample of semen.

NOTES ON DIAGNOSIS

Many investigators now emphasize the importance of subdividing MAGI into specific disease entities. These include acute bacterial prostatitis, chronic bacterial prostatitis, chronic abacterial prostatitis, seminal vesiculitis and epididymitis. Identification of the causative organism is necessary for effective drug therapy (Fair & Sharer, 1986). A close liaison should therefore be fostered with the genitourinary and microbiology departments for the proper evaluation of this group of patients.
       The diagnosis of MAGI should ideally be based upon the isolation of pathogenic organism(s) from one or more male accessory glands. In practice, this is often difficult (Comhaire et al., 1980) as the glands are not readily accessible for bacteriological examination. Indeed, many cases of MAGI are chronic and bacteriological examination is often negative. A further problem involves bacterial contamination of specimens taken from the upper urinary tract or urethra and infection in these sites must always be excluded.

1. History and physical signs

a.   Acute MAGI – this condition is often caused by a urinary tract infection or urethritis when symptoms and signs may be present. The presence of testicular and perineal pain, urinary urgency, hesitancy, diminished urinary stream, pain on ejaculation, with a tender swollen prostate or epididymis indicates spread of infection to the accessory glands. The seminal vesicles which lie lateral to the prostate are not normally palpable on rectal examination except when inflammed. Prostatic massage should not be performed in any patient suspected of having acute bacterial prostatitis as septicaemia often results. The clinical features are sufficiently characteristic to allow prompt diagnosis and treatment.

b. *Chronic MAGI* – A clinical history suggestive of chronic MAGI includes previous recurrent episodes of urinary tract infection or urethritis. In addition, aching pains may occur commonly referred to the suprapubic region, perineum, penis or testicles. Pains may also be associated with micturition and ejaculation. On urogenital examination there may be a urethral discharge or epididymal thickening. The prostate may be enlarged and boggy. It is however, not uncommon in the presence of a typical history of chronic MAGI to find no physical signs.

Recurrent urethral discharge in young men is a condition which is often misdiagnosed as 'chronic prostatitis'. Repeated sexually transmitted infections and reinfection from an untreated sexual partner need exclusion. Such men may occasionally have a urethral stricture which can be diagnosed by a urethrogram or urethrocystoscopy.

2. Prostatic fluid

Chronic bacterial prostatitis (CBP) is distinguished from abacterial prostatitis by laboratory tests. Expressed prostatic secretion (EPS) and urine samples should be examined microscopically and cultures performed for *T. vaginalis, mycoplasmas, C. trachomatis*, aerobic and anaerobic bacteria (see DeTure, 1985). Examination of prostatic fluid for *C. trachomatis* by tissue culture is often negative and detection by monoclonal antibody needs evaluation.

A method of localising infection in the lower urinary tract has been described by Meares and Stamey (1972).

1.   Clean glans with an antiseptic, rinse in sterile water and dry with a sterile gauze.

2.   Collect the first 5-10 ml of urine voided into a sterile container (VB1).

3.   A midstream urine sample is then collected (VB2).

4.   Prostatic massage is then performed and the EPS is collected and sent for gram stain and culture.

5.   After 4, collect a further 5-10 ml of urine (VB3).

A diagnosis of bacterial prostatitis can be made if the bacterial count of the EPS or VB3 are more than tenfold those in VB1 and VB2.

In chronic prostatitis there is usually over 80 WBC/HPF (EPS normally contains < 10 WBC/HPF). Bacterial cultures are necessary to distinguish bacterial from abacterial prostatitis.

Prostatdynia

Patients suffering with this condition have symptoms of prostatitis but clinical examination and EPS are normal. Other pathology such as urethritis, interstitial cystitis or neoplastic lesions of the bladder should be excluded.

3. Semen

a. Culture

Two important points should be borne in mind:

(i)   The mere presence of organisms in the ejaculate does not necessarily indicate an active infection. It is important to establish if such organisms are part of the normal flora or represent an active infection. To successfully distinguish these, quantitative culture techniques are usually necessary (De Ture, 1985; Weidner et al., 1985; Paulson and Leto, 1985).

(ii)   The diagnostic value of microbiological analyses of the ejaculate is limited by two factors. Firstly, as is the case with most comparable specimens, such as prostatic secretions, the ejaculate may be contaminated with other pathogens e.g. from the urethra; and secondly, some components of seminal fluid exert a bactericidal effect against gram positive bacteria and C. trachomatis (Wiedner et al., 1985).

Comhaire (1983) has suggested that the presence of 1×10^3 pathogenic or 1×10^4 non pathogenic bacteria/ml of semen is representative of an infection. However, the demarcation between pathogenic and non pathogenic organisms is contentious. Further research utilizing quantitative culture techniques is therefore necessary to clarify this issue.

b. Semen analysis

The relationship between a number of different organisms and semen characteristics is equivocal. For example, Grizard et al. (1985) suggested that a concentration of bacteria in semen of 1×10^4/ml adversely affected sperm motility and the number of abnormal forms. Recent work contradicts this – Naessens et al. (1986) could find no relationship between abnormal semen parameters and the presence of specific bacteria. To date, there would appear to be no distinct abnormality of the spermatozoa which would indicate a MAGI.

c. Number of white blood cells (WBC)

The presence of, or an increase in, the number of WBC in the ejaculate are thought to be representative of an infection (Weidner et al., 1985). However, there is controversial data on the relationship between the number of WBC and

MAGI. For example, Comhaire *et al.* (1980) showed that ejaculates with more than one million peroxidase positive leucocytes per ml represented significantly more pathogenic bacterial isolates than a group with less than 1 million peroxidase positive leucocytes per ml in their semen. This contrasts with the results of Berger *et al.* (1982), when microbiological studies of semen could not be correlated to the number of leucocytes in semen. A recent study by Monteiro *et al.*, (1987) could find no relationship between the number of WBC and urethral infection in semen donors.

Undoubtedly, the controversy regarding the relationship between seminal WBC and MAGI is partially a result of inadequate techniques to detect, classify and quantify these WBC. Very recently, accurate and reliable cell marker techniques, e.g. monoclonal antibodies, have been used to identify these WBC (El-Demiry *et al.* 1986). Future research into their nature and significance, as well as precursor spermatogenic cells, will rely on using these cell markers in conjunction with a systematic clinical evaluation.

d. Biochemistry

Recently, the traditional parameters of prostatic and seminal vesicle fluid e.g. acid phosphatase, fructose, and citric acid, as indicators of infection have been questioned (Grizard *et al.*, 1985). Interestingly, a multicentre study by the World Health Organization (WHO, 1987) has shown that the total output of citric acid in the ejaculate is probably the most reliable indicator of infection, i.e. levels below 10 mg/ml ejaculate were significantly related to infection. Other markers of infection are readily available, e.g. zinc levels in semen (Johnsen and Elisson, 1987).

Epididymo-orchitis

This condition is diagnosed clinically. In acute infection the patient is usually pyrexial with a unilateral tender swollen epididymis which may involve the testicle. Torsion of the testicle must always be considered. In men below the age of 35 sexually transmitted pathogens such as *C. trachomatis* are usually responsible but over this age urinary tract pathogens are increasingly involved (Grant *et al.* 1987). Berger *et al.* (1978) obtained aspirates from the epididymis to identify the aetiological agent. This procedure would be considered too traumatic in routine cases, therefore urethral swabs and midstream urine specimens should be cultured. In cases where sexually transmitted pathogens are isolated, sexual partners should be investigated and treated.

SUMMARY

Male accessory gland infection may have an important role in male infertility. Suspicion of this condition often comes from routine history taking and clinical examination. The diagnosis can be established by careful microscopic and bacteriological examination of expressed prostatic secretions and urine samples. Further studies are necessary to define which semen parameters indicate MAGI.

References

Berger, R.E., Alexander, E.R., Monda, G.B., Ansell, J., McCormick, G. and Holmes, K.K. (1978). Chlamydia trachomatis as a cause of acute idiopathic epidydimitis. *N. Engl. J. Med.*, **298**, 301–4

Berger, R.E., Karp, L.E., Williamson, R.A., Koehler, H., Moore, D.E. and Holmes, K.K. (1982). The relationship of pyospermia and seminal fluid bacteriology to sperm function as reflected in the sperm penetration assay. *Fertil. Steril.*, **37**, 557–64

Comhaire, F. (1983). Diagnosis and treatment of male adnexitis in relation to infertility. In Nigro-Vila (ed.) *Male Reproduction and Fertility.* pp. 265–72 (New York: Plenum Press)

Comhaire, F., Verschraegen, G. and Vermeulen, L. (1980). Diagnosis of accessory gland infection and its possible role in male infertility. *Int. J. Androl.*, **3**, 32–45

Comhaire, F.H., Rowe, P.J. and Farley, T.M.M. (1986). The effect of doxycline in infertile couples with male accessory gland infection: a double blind prospective study. *Int. J. Androl.*, **9**, 91–98

DeTure, F.A. (1985). The effects of lower urinary tract and reproductive organ infections on male infertility. In Keith, L.G., Berger, G.S. and Edelman, D.A. (eds.) *Infections in Reproductive Health (1) Common Infections.* pp. 267–82 (Lancaster: MTP Press)

El-Demiry, M.I.M., Hargreave, T.B., Busuttil, A., James, K. and Chisholm, G.D. (1986). Identifying leucocytes and leucocyte subpopulations in semen using monoclonal antibody probes. *Urology*, **28**, 492–6

Fair, W.R. and Sharer, W. (1986). Prostatitis. In Blandy, J.P. and Lytton, B. (eds.) *The Prostate.* pp. 33–50. (London: Butterworth)

Grant, J.B.F., Costello, C.B., Sequeira, P.J.L. and Blacklock, N.J. (1987). The role of Chlamydia trachomatis in epididymitis. *Br. J. Urol.*, **60**, 355–9

Grizard, G., Janny, L., Hermabessiere, J., Sirot, J. and Boucher, D. (1985). Seminal biochemistry and sperm characteristics in infertile men with bacteria in ejaculate. *Arch. Androl.*, **15**, 181–6

Johnsen, O and Eliasson, R. (1987). Evaluation of a commercially available kit for the colorimetric determination of zinc in human seminal plasma. *Int. J. Androl.*, **10**, 435–40

Keith, L.G., Berger, G.S. and Edelman, D.A. (eds)(1985a). *Infections in Reproductive Health (I) Common Infections.* p. 375. (Lancaster: MTP Press)

Keith, L.G., Berger, G.S. and Edelman, D.A. (eds)(1985b). *Infections in Reproductive Health (II) Uncommon Infections and Special Topics.* p. 393. (Lancaster: MTP Press)

Meares, E.M. and Stamey, T.A. (1972). The diagnosis and management of bacterial prostatitis. *Br. J. Urol.*, **44**, 175–9

Monteiro, E.F., Spencer, R.C., Kinghorn, G.R.Y., Barratt, C.L.R., Cooke, S. and Cooke, I.D. (1987). Sexually transmitted disease in potential semen donors. *Br. Med. J.*, **295**, 415

Naessens, A., Foulon, W., Debrucker, P., Devroey, P. and Lauwers, S. (1986). Recovery of microorganisms in semen and relationship to semen evaluation. *Fertil. Steril.* **45**, 101–5

Paulson, J.D. and Leto, S. (1985). The reproductive effects of microorganisms in semen. In Keith, L.G., Berger, G.S. and Edelman, D.A. (eds.) *Infections in Reproductive Health (1) Common Infections.* pp. 355–62. (Lancaster: MTP Press)

Weidner, W., Krause, W. and Brunner, H. (1985). The role of mycoplasmas and chlamydiae in infertility. In Keith, L.G., Berger, G.S. and Edelman, D.A. (eds.) *Infections in Reproductive Health (1) Common Infections.* pp. 323–36. (Lancaster: MTP Press)

World Health Organization (1987). Towards more objectivity in diagnosis and management of male fertility. Supplement 7 *Int. J. Androl.* Vol. 10

10
DEVELOPMENT OF IN VITRO SYSTEMS FOR THE DIAGNOSIS OF HUMAN SPERM FUNCTION

R.J. Aitken, D.S. Irvine, J.S. Clarkson and D.W. Richardson

INTRODUCTION

The traditional criteria of semen quality are based upon a descriptive assessment of the semen in terms of its volume, biochemical markers of prostate and seminal vesicle function and the concentration, motility and morphology of the spermatozoa. The shortcomings of such an approach have been repeatedly emphasized however, and are reflected by the fact that men with pathological semen profiles have been consistently observed in surveys of the normal fertile population (MacLeod, 1971). Furthermore patients, with seriously defective spermatozoa and yet perfectly normal semen profiles, have been detected within the cohort of couples exhibiting unexplained infertility (Aitken *et al.*, 1982a). These observations, together with the fact that pregnancies have been reported when the sperm count has been lowered to less than 5×10^6/ml by exogenous steroid therapy (Barfield *et al.*, 1979), suggest that it is not so much the number of gametes which is the critical determinant of male infertility, but their functional competence. Such reasoning has led to the development of a new generation of diagnostic tests for male fertility which focus on the biological functions of the spermatozoa rather than their number or appearance. It is the purpose of this chapter to review the nature and application of such tests and consider their place in the diagnosis of male fertility.

SPERM MOVEMENT AND CERVICAL MUCUS PENETRATION

Recent advances in our understanding of the factors regulating sperm-cervical mucus interaction have stemmed from the widespread use of objective methods to quantitate the movement characteristics of human spermatozoa, the refinement of Kremer-type tests to quantitate the degree of sperm penetration and the development of rapid LH radioimmunoassays to time the cervical mucus aspiration with greater accuracy (Aitken, Warner and Reid, 1986).

The simplest means of quantifying the movement characteristics of human spermatozoa is by time exposure photomicrography. With this technique the spermatozoa are photographed at 37°C, under dark field illumination using an exposure time of 1 s (Overstreet *et al.*, 1979; Aitken *et al.*, 1982 a,b,c, 1985). The path travelled by the sperm head is visualized as a track on the photomicrograph from which direct measurements can be made of specific aspects of sperm movement. For example, the length of each track will give the

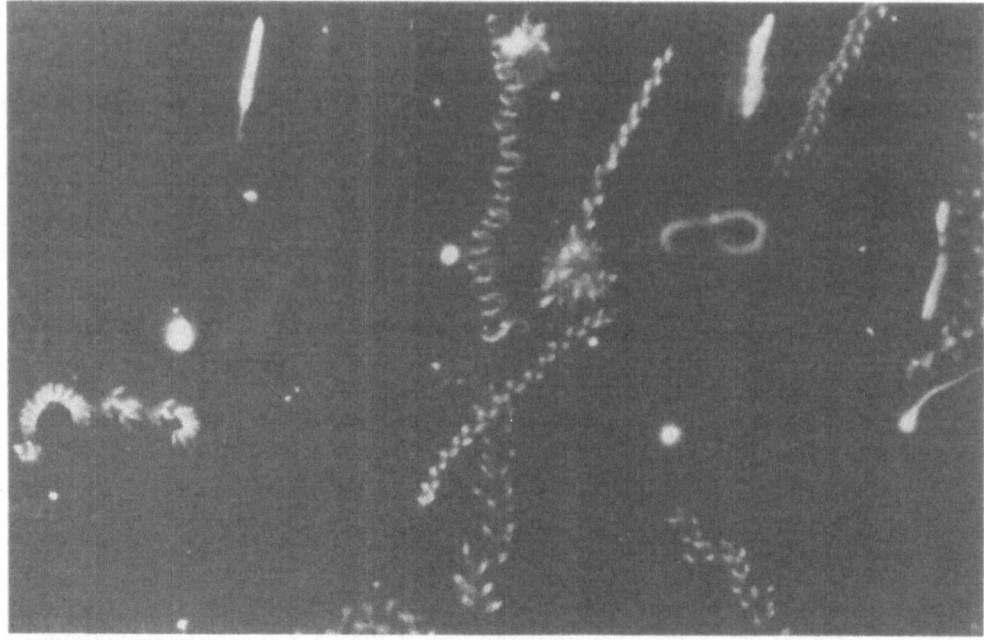

Figure 10.1 Dark field time exposure photomicrography of human sperm movement.

linear velocity of forward progression, the width of each track will give the amplitude of lateral sperm head displacement, and the number of successive head images will provide information on the frequency of sperm head rotation (Figure 10.1). The apparatus for obtaining the photomicrographs is very inexpensive and the technique itself is rapid and accurate. The major defect of this method is that it is ineffective with samples contaminated with extraneous cells or debris, which scatter light and hinder resolution of the spermatozoa. Furthermore, it is ineffective with samples exhibiting severe asthenozoospermia, when the spermatozoa are so poorly motile that they do not leave an adequate image with an exposure time as short as 1 s. A solution to this problem is to use videomicrography or cinematography, both of which are capable of generating data on the flagellar wave form, in addition to the movement of the sperm head (David, Serres and Jouannet, 1981). Whether the additional expense and time required to make optimal use of such systems are cost-effective, in terms of the clinical diagnosis male fertility, has yet to be determined. A pointer to the future is the recent introduction of fully automated video analysis systems such as 'Cell

Soft' which generate data on mean velocity, amplitude of lateral sperm head displacement, beat frequency, and the linearity of progression in a fraction of the time required by the above techniques. Although such systems are currently extremely expensive they will undoubtedly find widespread application in the future.

Table 10.1 Multiple regression of sperm density in human cervical mucus on the movement characteristics of human spermatozoa (n = 37; Aitken *et al.*, 1986)

Variable	Multiple R	R^2	R^2 Change	B*	β*
Sperm density (10^6/ml)	0.782	0.611	0.611	0.124	0.924
Motility (%)	0.865	0.748	0.137	0.412	0.361
Progressive rolling (%)[+]	0.912	0.831	0.082	0.229	0.228
Progressive, amplitude < 10 μm (%)[+]	0.932	0.868	0.037	-0.582	-0.256
Yawing (%)	0.944	0.891	0.02	−0.381	−0.160
Constant (A)				20.197	

B = unstandardized regression coefficient; β = standardized regression coefficient, reflecting relative contribution of each variable to the overall regression equation.
[+] Progressive = linear velocity of > 25 μm/sec:; amplitude = amplitude of lateral sperm head displacement.

Table 10.2 Multiple regression of sperm density in human cervical mucus on the movement characteristics of human spermatozoa (n = 37; Aitken *et al.*, 1986)

Variable	Multiple R	R^2	R^2 Change	B*	β*
Progressive, amplitude < μm (%)[+]	0.522	0.272	0.272	-2.102	-0.553
Yawing (%)	0.654	0.428	0.156	-1.978	-0.497
Progressive, mean velocity (μm/sec)[+]	0.752	0.565	0.137	2.154	0.228
Progressive, rolling (%)[+]	0.779	0.608	0.043	0.398	0.236
Motility (%)	0.807	0.651	0.043	0.471	0.247
Constant				132.860	

B = unstandardized regression coefficient; β = standardized regression coefficient, reflecting relative contribution of each variable to the overall regression equation.

The interaction between spermatozoa and cervical mucus has been quantified using variations of the Kremer-test, such as the SPT scoring system introduced by Pandya *et al.* (1986) or the calculation of Percentage Successful Collisions (PSC) described by Katz, Overstreet and Hanson (1980). The PSC test involves calculation of the number of spermatozoa penetrating the cervical mucus in 30 min and expression of the result as a percentage of the total number of spermatozoa colliding with the cervical mucus interface over the same time period. The latter is determined from data describing the concentration of motile sperm cells and their total mean velocity (Katz *et al.*, 1980). Using this technique we have been able to carry out detailed quantitative analyses of the factors determining the success of sperm-cervical mucus interaction in couples with otherwise unexplained infertility (Aitken *et al.*, 1986).

In this cohort of patients, simultaneous assessment of sperm penetration into the female partner's cervical mucus and, as a positive control, bovine cervical mucus, revealed a very high correlation (r = 0.931) between these two sets of measurements. This result suggested that it is the quality of the spermatozoa rather than the mucus itself which, in general, determines the success of sperm penetration. Multiple regression analyses using the concentration of spermatozoa penetrating the cervical mucus in unit time as the dependent variable and the movement characteristics of the spermatozoa as the independent variables, gave a multiple R value of 0.944 after five criteria of sperm quality had been incorporated into the regression equation. This result indicated that 89% of the variation in cervical mucus penetration could be explained by variations in the movement characteristics exhibited by the spermatozoa (Aitken *et al.*, 1986; Table 10.1). The first incorporated and most significant variables entered into this equation (sperm density and motility) simply reflect the expected impact of the motile sperm concentration on the frequency of collisions between spermatozoa and the cervical mucus interface (Mortimer, Pandya and Sawers, 1986), i.e. the higher the total number of spermatozoa colliding with the cervical mucus interface, the higher the chances of penetration. Through the use of the PSC system we can also examine those attributes of sperm movement which determine whether a spermatozoon colliding with the mucus interface is likely to achieve penetration, since this method of expressing the results incorporates a measure of collision frequency. When multiple regression analysis was performed using the PSC values as the dependent variable, five aspects of sperm movement were drawn into the regression equation on the basis of which 65% of the variability in mucus penetration could be explained (Table 10.2). The most significant movement characteristic identified in this study was the percentage of progressive spermatozoa exhibiting an amplitude of lateral sperm head displacement of less than 10 μm, which was negatively correlated with mucus penetration. Hence a spermatozoon colliding with the cervical mucus interface will achieve penetration only if it possesses an adequate degree of lateral sperm head displacement.

Independent studies on separate groups of patients (Aitken, 1985; Mortimer *et al.*, 1986) have also emphasized the importance of lateral sperm head displacement in achieving penetration of human cervical mucus. The higher the proportion of cells exhibiting negligible (< 4.5 μm) lateral displacement, the lower the capacity of the sample for mucus penetration. Both Feneux *et al.* (1985) and ourselves (Aitken *et al.*, 1985, 1986) have independently identified patients whose infertility appears to stem from the fact that their spermatozoa are incapable of penetrating cervical mucus, because of inadequacies in the degree of lateral sperm head displacement. Significantly, many of these patients have apparently normal semen profiles and would have been diagnosed as fertile if objective techniques had not been used to assess the movement characteristics of their spermatozoa.

This correlation between lateral sperm head displacement and cervical mucus penetration may reflect a physical need for lateral sperm movements, in order to insinuate the sperm head into the channels between the cervical mucin chains. Alternatively, the actual displacement of the sperm head may simply be of value in reflecting the efficiency of the flagellar wave form. The amplitude of lateral sperm head displacement is positively correlated with the size of the flagellar beating envelope (David, Serres and Jouannet, 1981). For spermatozoa arriving at the cervical mucus interface the forward thrust driving the sperm head into the mucus will be proportional to the amplitude of the flagellar wave and hence the degree of lateral displacement exhibited by the sperm head. Clearly, it is now important that we establish which intracellular factors regulate the amplitude of the flagellar wave form, in order to determine the biochemical basis for the aberrant form of motility described above.

SPERM-ZONA INTERACTION

Cervical mucus penetration is not the only aspect of sperm function which is dependent upon the shearing forces generated by sperm motility. Penetration of the zona pellucida is a major obstacle to fertilization which involves aspects of cell recognition as well as sperm movement. Zona penetration is also favoured by flagellar beats of large amplitude and in many subhuman species, such as the mouse, hamster, guinea pig and marmoset monkey, capacitation of the spermatozoa is associated with a change in the pattern of sperm motility to a hyperactivated form, which is characterized by asymmetric flagellar beats of large amplitude (Uanagimachi, 1981). Although no direct equivalent of 'hyperactivated' motility has been observed with human spermatozoa, the same general relationship between the amplitude of the flagellar waveform and the efficiency of zona penetration appears to exist. Hence in a recent study by Jeulin *et al.* (1986) concerning the sperm factors responsible for failure of human *in vitro* fertilization, a poor amplitude of lateral sperm head displacement was again shown to be a critical determinant. In view of the importance of this specific aspect of sperm movement to the penetration of both cervical mucus and the zona pellucida it is not surprising that Hull *et al.* (1984) have observed a correlation between the outcome of the postcoital test and fertilization *in vitro*.

These findings are of practical importance since they suggest that direct assessments of sperm movement or cervical mucus penetration should give an accurate indication of the competence of a sperm sample to achieve penetration of the zona pellucida. This aspect of sperm function is extremely difficult to assess directly in view of the scarcity of human zona material and the lack of an appropriate surrogate that might be used for routine screening purposes. Although the use of salt-stored human zonae (Yanagimachi *et al.*, 1979) goes some way towards solving some of the practical and ethical problems of establishing a bioassay for sperm-zona interaction, the limited availability of human material remains a difficult problem.

SPERM–OOCYTE INTERACTION

The above problems have been largely overcome in establishing a bioassay to assess the competence of human spermatozoa to fuse with the vitelline membrane of the oocyte. The discovery by Yanagimachi, Yanagimachi and Rocherts (1976) that zona-free hamster oocytes are uniquely susceptible to penetration by human spermatozoa has provided a surrogate for the human oocyte, suitable for the development of a routine diagnostic test. The fusion between human spermatozoa and the vitelline membrane of the hamster oocyte reflects the homologous situation in that this process is initiated by the vitelline membrane over-lying the equatorial segment of acrosome reacted spermatozoa. Penetration of zona-free hamster oocytes therefore provides important information on a range of human sperm function including their ability to capacitate and acrosome react *in vitro*, generate a fusogenic equatorial segment, fuse with the vitelline membrane of the oocyte and undergo nuclear decondensation. Despite the fact that a number of important sperm functions are not assessed by this bioassay, notably those associated with the ascent of the female reproductive tract and zona penetration, correlations have been repeatedly described between the incidence of male infertility and the relative ability of spermatozoa to penetrate zona-free hamster oocytes (Rogers, 1985; Aitken, 1986). Since many of the functions which are not assessed by the hamster oocyte assay are heavily dependent upon sperm motility, it is not surprising that the most complete and accurate assessments of sperm function have come from studies involving the simultaneous assessment of sperm movement characteristics and zona-free hamster oocyte penetration (Aitken et al, 1984; Aitken, 1985; Irvine and Aitken, 1986a).

This association was, for example, recently demonstrated in a prospective study of patients exhibiting a mean ($\pm$ SEM) of 4.7 $\pm$ 0.6 years infertility associated with oligozoospermia (Aitken, 1985). The female partners of these couples were all normal, according to a variety of criteria including diagnostic laparoscopy, while the male partners presented with sperm counts consistently below 20×10^6/ml. A single semen specimen from each of the 27 patients was examined at the beginning of the study to assess the movement characteristics of the spermatozoa and their capacity for hamster oocyte penetration. They were then followed up for a period of 4.2 ± 1.1 years, during which time 25.9% of the couples spontaneously achieved a pregnancy. A multivariate discriminant analysis was subsequently performed to determine which of the various criteria of semen ability, assessed at the initiation of the study, most accurately predicted the later incidence of pregnancy. A total of seven variables was selected in this analysis (Table 10.3) four of which were positively related to fertility (morphology, velocity, hamster oocyte penetration and the proportion of progressive, straight swimming spermatozoa) with sperm velocity and hamster oocyte penetration possessing the largest discriminant function coefficients, i.e. these variables contributed the greatest amount of information to the overall accuracy of the classification. Three variables were identified with a negative association with fertility, the most significant factor being the proportion of the spermatozoa with an amplitude of lateral sperm head displacement of less than 10 mm. Samples were assessed as 'fertile' or 'infertile' on the basis of the above variables with an accuracy of 85.2%. This discrimination is, of course, optimized for this particular data set, and will have to be repeated on independent groups of oligozoospermic men. Nevertheless, the results are extremely encouraging and emphasize the value of coupling assessments of sperm movement to the outcome of hamster oocyte assay. In particular, the significance of assessing the amplitude of lateral head displacement was again emphasized by these studies, presumably reflecting the significance of this aspect of sperm movement in achieving those functions which are heavily dependent on sperm motility (such as cervical mucus penetration or interaction with the zona pellucida) which are not assessed by the hamster oocyte penetration test.

Table 10.3 Variables used to discriminate fertile from infertile oligozoospermic men (Aitken, 1985)

Variables	Standardized discriminant function coefficients
Normal morphology	0.37461
Velocity	0.70075
*Ah < 10 μm (10^6/ml)	-1.24570
Hamster oocyte penetration (%)	0.67765
Progressive, straight swimming (%)	0.52427
+Log progressive, Ah 10 μm (%)	-0.37791
Log sperm concentration (10^6/ml)	-0.46905

*Ah = amplitude of lateral sperm head displacement
+Progressive = velocity of > 25 μm/sec

105

One of the inherent defects in a study with the above design is that the assessments of sperm function are carried out on a different sample from that which ultimately establishes a pregnancy. Because of the significant variation in sperm function which is known to occur between ejaculates from the same donor (Aitken and Elton, 1986), there is bound to be some inaccuracy in predicting the fertility of an individual from the attributes of a single sample. Further inaccuracy will also be introduced because of variations in the fertility of the female partners, which were not detected in the routine work-up of each couple. Both of these sources of variation have been overcome through the analyses of samples employed in an AID clinic. In this study (Irvine and Aitken, 1986a,b) analyses of sperm movement, hamster oocyte penetration, ATP content and the conventional semen profile, were carried out on the same sample that was subsequently used to inseminate at least four independent recipients. A total of 48 cryostored ejaculates were analysed in this way, of which 27 established a pregnancy. When the mean values obtained for each criterion of semen quality were compared between samples which did or did not establish a pregnancy, only three variables were found to show significant differences. These were the concentration of motile cells inseminated and the outcome of the zona-free hamster egg penetration test expressed in two different ways (percentage of hamster oocytes penetrated and mean number of spermatozoa penetrating each oocyte).

Table10. 4 Variables used to discriminate successful from unsuccessful samples within the context of an AID programme

Variable	Standardized discriminant function coefficients
Concentration of motile spermatozoa $(10^6/\text{ml})$	0.056024
Mean velocity (μm/sec)	0.64552
Amplitude of lateral head displacement < 4.5 μm (%)	-4.50812
Frequency of head rotation of progressive* spermatozoa (μm/sec)	-1.02452
Percentage of progressive* rolling, spermatozoa	-4.39228
Percentage of progressive* yawing spermatozoa	-0.51156

*Progressive = velocity of > 25 μm/sec

When the movement characteristics of the spermatozoa were fed into a multivariate discriminant analyses six variables were identified which permitted a prediction of the relative fertility of these AID samples with an overall accuracy of 72.9%. These variables are listed in Table 10.4. The most important criterion was the proportion of spermatozoa exhibiting a low amplitude of lateral sperm head displacement (Ah < 4.5 μm), which was negatively correlated with fertility. This finding is again in accord with the data presented above indicating that sperm functions dependent on the shearing forces generated by sperm motility are positively correlated with an adequate degree of lateral sperm head displacement.

Of the other variables identified, the concentration of motile spermatozoa inseminated and their total mean velocity were both positively correlated with fertility, as might be expected. In contrast, variables describing the attributes of that subpopulation of spermatozoa exhibiting very high velocities, 25 μm/s, were negatively associated with fertility. A negative correlation between high sperm velocities and the fertilizing capacity of human spermatozoa has been reported in a number of independent studies both *in vivo* (Aitken *et al.*, 1984a; Irvine and Aitken 1986a,b) and *in vitro* (Cohen *et al.*, 1982; Aitken *et al.*, 1983). It is possible that this negative correlation is due to the fact that defective spermatozoa exhibiting low amplitudes of lateral sperm head displacement tend to exhibit high forward velocities. Alternatively, we have previously observed a significant negative correlation between the velocity of human spermatozoa and the intracellular concentration of ATP ($r = 0.361$, $p = 0.01$, $n = 48$). It is therefore possible that samples exhibiting high velocities progressively utilize more ATP for movement than can be generated by processes such as glycolysis. As a result, the steady state levels of ATP might gradually decline and important ATP-dependent cellular processes such as calcium ion extrusion (Irvine and Aitken, 1986c) would then suffer, leading to a loss of cell viability.

If these movement characteristics were supplemented with data describing capacity of human spermatozoa for hamster oocyte penetration, subsequent discriminant analysis managed to classify the fertile and the infertile AID samples, with an overall accuracy of 81.25% (Irvine and Aitken, 1986a,b). These findings are of clinical importance in predicting the likely fertility of samples submitted to an AID programme. In addition they emphasize the prognostic value of simultaneously evaluating both sperm movement and hamster oocyte penetration, since these techniques target separate, complementary aspects of sperm function.

CONCLUSIONS

In conclusion, a variety of new diagnostic tests have been developed which focus upon the dynamics of sperm function rather than the traditional, descriptive, semen profile. These *in vitro* bioassays are capable of generating objective information on the capacity of human spermatozoa for cervical mucus penetration, capacitation, the acrosome reaction and sperm-oocyte fusion. Aspects of sperm behaviour which are not directly assessed by these systems, particularly those dependent on motility such as sperm migration through the female reproductive tract or sperm-zona interaction, can be indirectly evaluated through the objective measurement of sperm movement. Both prospective and retrospective studies employing these diagnostic techniques have shown a high correlation with fertility *in vivo*, achieving classifications of fertility which exhibit an accuracy of around 80-85%.

The future of male fertility diagnosis now depends upon the use of these bioassays to determine the underlying nature of the lesions present in the spermatozoa. In the case of sperm movement, for example, we now need to determine the nature of the intracellular factors determining the amplitude of the flagellar wave, possibly using demembranated sperm models which can be reactivated by ATP. Furthermore, failures of sperm-oocyte fusion in the hamster-oocyte system can now be analysed to determine the nature of the defects present in the plasma membrane. Existing studies have already shown that such defects are downstream from the calcium influx induced by ionophores such as A23187 (Aitken *et al.*, 1984b) and are frequently associated with the excessive generation of reactive oxygen species by the spermatozoa. By analysing the mechanism by which such reactive oxygen species are generated and their influence on the composition and properties of the sperm plasma membrane, we can begin to unravel the aetiology of pathological sperm function and take a rational approach towards the development of appropriate methods of therapy.

References

Aitken, R.J. (1985). Diagnostic value of the zona-free hamster oocyte penetration test and sperm movement characteristics in oligozoospermia. *Int. J. Androl.*, **8**, 348-56

Aitken, R.J. (1986). The zona-free hamster oocyte penetration test and the diagnosis of male fertility. *Int. J. Androl.*, Suppl. 6

Aitken, R.J. and Elton, R.A. (1986). Quantitative analysis of sperm-egg interaction in the zona-free hamster egg penetration test. *Int. J. Androl.*, Suppl. 6, 14-30

Aitken, R.J., Best, F.S.M., Richardson, D.W. *et al.* (1982a). An analysis of sperm function in cases of unexplained infertility: conventional criteria, movement characteristics and fertilizing capacity. *Fertil. Steril.*, 38, 212-21

Aitken, R.J., Best, F.S.M., Richardson, D.W. *et al.* (1982b). An analysis of semen quality and sperm function in cases of oligozoospermia. *Fertil. Steril.*, **38**, 705-14

Aitken, R.J., Best, F.S.M., Richardson, D.W. *et al.* (1982c). The correlates of fertilizing capacity in normal fertile men. *Fertil. Steril.*, 38, 68-76

Aitken, R.J., Warner, P., Best, F.S.M. *et al.* (1983). The predictability of subnormal penetrating capacity of sperm in cases of unexplained infertility. *Int. J. Androl.*, 6, 212-20

Aitken, R.J., Best, F.S.M., Warner, P. and Templeton, A.A. (1984a). A prospective study of the relationship between semen quality and fertility in cases of unexplained infertility. *J. Androl.*, 5, 297-303

Aitken, R.J., Ross, A., Hargreave, T. *et al.* (1984b). Analysis of human sperm function following exposure to the ionophore A23187: comparison of normospermic and oligozoospermic men. *J. Androl.*, **5**, 321-9

Aitken, R.J., Sutton, M., Warner, P. and Richardson, D.W. (1985). Relationship between the movement characteristics of human spermatozoa and their ability to penetrate cervical mucus and zona-free hamster oocytes. *J. Reprod. Fertil.*, **73**, 441-9

Aitken, R.J., Warner, P.E. and Reid, C. (1986). Factors influencing the success of sperm-cervical mucus interaction in patients exhibiting unexplained infertility. *J. Androl.*, **7**, 3-10

Barfield, A., Melo, J., Coutinho, E. *et al.* (1979). Pregnancies associated with sperm concentrations below 10 million/ml in clinical studies of a potential male contraceptive method, monthly depot medroxyprogesterone acetate and testosterone esters. *Contraception*, **10**, 121-7

Cohen, J., Mooyaart, M., Vreeburg, J.T.M. and Zeilmaker, G.H. (1982). Fertilization of hamster ova by human spermatozoa in relation to other semen parameters. *Int. J. Androl.*, **5**, ?10-15

David, G., Serres, C. and Jouannet, P. (1981). Kinematics of human spermatozoa. *Gamete Res.*, **4**, 83-95

Feneux, D., Serres, C. and Jounnaet, P. (1985). Sliding spermatozoa: a dyskinesia responsible for human infertility? *Fertil. Steril.*, **44**, 508-11

Hull, M.G.R., McLeod, F.N., Joyce, D.N. *et al.* (1984). Human *in vitro* fertilization, in vivo penetration of cervical mucus and unexplained infertility. *Lancet*, **2**, 245-8

Irvine, D.S. and Aitken, R.J. (1986a). Clinical evaluation of the zona-free hamster egg penetration test in the management of the infertile couple. Prospective and retrospective studies. *Int. J. Androl.*, Suppl.6, 97-112

Irvine, D.S. and Aitken, R.J. (1986b). Predictive value of *in vitro* sperm function tests in the context of an AID service. *Human Reprod.*, **1**, 539-45

Irvine, D.S. nd Aitken, R.J. (1986c). Measurement of intracellular calcium in human spermatozoa. *Gamete Res.*, **15**, 52-72

Jeulin, C., Feneux, D., Serres, C. *et al.*, (1986). Sperm factors related to failure of human *in vitro* fertilization. *J. Reprod. Fertil.*, **76**, 735-44

Katz, D.F.R. and Overstreet, J.W. (1981). Sperm motility assessment by videomicrography. *Fertil. Steril.*, **35**, 188-93

Katz, D.F., Overstreet, J.W. and Hanson, F.W. (1980). A new quantitative test for sperm penetration into cervical mucus. *Fertil. Steril.*, **33**, 179-86

MacLeod, J. (1971). Human male infertility. *Obstet. Gynaecol. Survey*, **26**, 335-51

Mortimer, D., Pandya, I.J. and Sawers, R.S. (1986). Relationship between human sperm motility characteristics and sperm penetration into human cervical mucus *in vitro*. *J. Reprod. Fertil.*, **78**, 93-102

Overstreet, J.W., Katz, D.F., Hanson, F.W. and Fonseca, J.R. (1979). A simple inexpensive method for objective assessment of human sperm movement characteristics. *Fertil. Steril.*, **31**, 162-72

Pandya, I.J., Mortimer, D. and Sawers, R.S. (1986). A standardized approach for evaluating the penetration of human spermatozoa into cervical mucus *in vitro*. *Fertil. Steril.*, **45**, 357-65

Rogers, B.J. (1985). The sperm penetration assay: Its usefulness re-evaluated. *Fertil. Steril.*, **43**, 821-40

Yanagimachi, R. (1981). Mechanisms of fertilization in mammals. In Mastrianni, L. Jnr. and Biggers, J. D. (eds.) Fertilization and embryonic development *in vitro*. pp. 82-155. (New York, London: Plenum Press)

Yanagimachi, R., Yanagimachi, H. and Rogers, B.J. (1976). The use of zona-free animal ova test system for the assessment of the fertilizing capacity of human spermatozoa. *Biol. Reprod.,* **15,** 471-76

Yanagimachi, R., Lopata, A., Odom, C.B. *et al.* (1979). Retention of biologic characteristics of zona pellucida in highly concentrated salt solution: the use of salt-stored eggs for assessing the fertilizing capacity of spermatozoa. *Fertil. Steril.,* **31,** 562-74

DISCUSSION

Question: We are currently setting up the Hamster Penetration Test (HPT); so far, we have not found any cumulus masses in the animals' oviducts, how often does this problem occur?

Aitken: Never. The animals always have cumulus masses. The critical thing is to use mature hamsters who are stimulated with large doses of gonadotrophins (up to 60 iu per animal).

Question: What is the importance of enzyme digestion by the spermatozoa in zona penetration?

Aitken: There are three components to zona penetration: (1) recognition – the sperm cell has to recognize the surface of the zona pellucida; (2) acrosome reaction – which is thought to release hydrolytic enzymes (e.g. acrosin) in order to effect proteolytic cleavage of the zona pellucida, and (3) spermatozoa motility – where the degree of lateral sperm head displacement is critical.

Question: As the acrosome reaction normally occurs in the vicinity of the zona pellucida, have the human spermatozoa that penetrate zona free hamster eggs undergone the acrosome reaction?

Aitken: Yes. In the normal biological situation, the spermatozoa binds to the zona pellucida, undergoes the acrosome reaction and penetrates. In the HPT, there is no zona pellucida, but this does not mean that the spermatozoa are not acrosome reacted, they are spontaneously undergoing a low level of acrosome reaction. If there is no stimulus to promote the acrosome reaction, e.g. zona pellucida, the penetration rates are low. If a stimulus for inducing the acrosome reaction is added (e.g. A23187) then penetration levels are very much higher (Aitken, R.J., Ross, A., Hargreave, T., Richardson, D. and Best F., 1984, *J. Androl.,* 5, 321–329).

Question: Sperm penetration of bovine cervical mucus may not be an adequate test of sperm function – for example with spermatozoa posessing a coating of surface-bound antibody, on the surface penetration of bovine mucus is not impaired.

Aitken: There is data supporting the opposite view. Studies have shown that sperm coated with antisperm IgA exhibit the same inhibition to penetration, as when human mucus was used. (Mangione, C.M., Medley, N.E. and Menge, A.C., 1981, *Int. J. Fert.*, 26, 20–24).

Question: Is there any correlation between penetration of cervical mucus and the hamster eggs?

Aitken: Yes. We have published two papers on this. (Aitken, R.J., Warner, P.E. and Reid, C. 1986, *J Androl.*, 7, 3–10; Aitken, R.J., Sutton, M., Warner, P. and Richardson, D.W. 1985, *J. Reprod. Fert.*, 73, 441–449). However, we don't understand why there is such a correlation as penetration of hamster eggs is not dependent upon motility of the spermatozoa.

Question: Is there an upper limit of normal for lateral head displacement?

Aitken: If measurements are made in semen, (those which are important when penetrating cervical mucus) then a displacement of less than 5 μm has discriminating value – the optimum would be 6–7 μm. When the spermatozoa are washed and incubated *in vitro* there is an increase in velocity and amplitude of displacement, at this moment we find a negative correlation between lateral head displacement and oocyte fusion – for example – a displacement of 10 μm in washed spermatozoa is negatively correlated to oocyte fusion. Therefore there is an optimal range of 6–7 μm.

Question: Have you correlated the use of hyperosmotic incubation medium with the use of A23187 with regard to the predictive power of the HPT?

Aitken: Yes, we have studied this in many groups of patients. Hyperosmotic medium strips decapacitation factors off the sperm surface, but is much less efficient at stimulating fusion than the A23187. Studies in progress suggest that the A23187 system has a great deal of discriminating power, and is a much more sensitive system.

Question: In some studies the outcome of conventional HPT does not show a good correlation with the human IVF system – any comments? (Rudak, E., Dor, J. Nebel, L., Maschiach, S. and Goldman, B. 1986, *Int. J. Androl.*, 6, 131–142).

Aitken: In our studies so far, none of the men who scored 0% penetration in the presence of A23187 fertilized a human egg, however, when we ran the conventional HPT or the hyperosmotic system some men scored 0 and went on to achieve a pregnancy.

11
THE FUTURE

I.D. Cooke

Using the information presented in the foregoing chapters it may be possible to look to the future in an attempt to see how infertility practice in the male may develop.

After a couple has been seen and their histories obtained, those data may be input directly by the physician into the preprogrammed computer while the patients undress. After physical examination similarly the next data set may be input. When the semen analyses have been completed the data may be entered directly from the laboratory and an appropriate diagnosis on the semen characteristics offered. The networked information from clinical and laboratory sources are then linked to provide a logical diagnosis with any errors or omissions highlighted to obtain consistency in investigation and clinical conclusion. At that time a report may be automatically prepared for the referring doctor. According to the nature of the infertility, whether it is primary or secondary, its duration and diagnosis, a cumulative conception curve may be generated to offer a prognosis and aid discussion and counselling with the patient. The couple will of course be more accurately assessed if the same process has been effected for the female partner and a cumulative conception rate prepared combining that for each individual's diagnosis. The shape of the curve and their position on that curve, particularly if a plateau has been reached will determine the advice offered.

Surgical exploration of the scrotum in azoospermia is likely to be recommended for diagnosis where plasma FSH estimation shows no elevation indicative of Sertoli cell damage and no elevated antisperm antibody titres suggesting immunological impairment of sperm surface membranes. Perhaps embolization will make varicoceles relatively easy to treat by the intervention radiologist.

There will be a substantial number of men however who have poor semen characteristics and will need to decide between *in vitro* fertilization and donor insemination after appropriate counselling. Further assessment of a compromised semen using computerized motility appraisal to evaluate the degree of lateral head displacement may give an indicator of likely fertilizing capacity and suggest perseverance or recourse to donor insemination after the requisite counselling of the couple. If this latter technique is readily available the data may be available initially to guide discussion.

If *in vitro* fertilization is readily available then homologous human test fertilization may be superior to a heterologous system such as the zona free hamster egg penetration test, although compromise of oocyte quality in the female partner may obscure the interpretability of the results.

Follicle growth may be abnormal in the presence of a compromised female oocyte so counselling may be indicated early and again suggest an attempt at homologous fertilization. This would assess oocyte fertilizability when there was a predictably good sperm fertilizing capacity. Where oocyte quality is compromised a donor oocyte may be required. Such routes to donor gamete usage may well remove considerable anxiety on the part of the couple and facilitate an early decision to use a donor.

Computer matching of donor and male partner characteristics would simplify screening of the donor bank and ensure that all choices were scrutinized. Similarly regular updating of pregnancy rates and donor stocks could readily be carried out aiding the elimination of samples of donors having sub optimal pregnancy rates and rapidly notifying the number of pregnancies and cycles in which a specific donor has been used. As data increase, cumulative conception curves can be generated as quality control of the bank function. In this way surveillance would be maintained and it would be known as early as possible when prospects of pregnancy calculated from a pregnancy rate per cycle became insupportably low. A similar approach to a donor bank would be predicted if the vitrification of oocytes ultimately yield good post-thaw fertilizability. Then a similar system of screening, banking, counselling, matching and data analysis for optimization could be applied. Where homologous test fertilization fails and the offer of donor gametes is declined or when donor gametes fail to achieve a pregnancy, acceptance of the infertility would be counselled. This would reduce the time taken to achieve a definite end point and reduce the prolonged waiting which so many couples experience. By computerization of semen anlysis it will be possible in due course routinely to assess lateral head displacement, for example in an initial sample and correlation with outcome (including of course the female factor) may estimate the usefulness of this parameter.

The use of the computer is not in itself modish but is rather a reflection of the clearer thought and systematic assessment that has allowed the development of a logical investigation and assessment of outcome. Thus a clearer evaluation of efficacy of any treatment may be obtained by reference to treatment independent conception rates, simplifying advice and avoiding the waste of time implicit in ineffectual remedies. Progress in the management of male infertility requires careful data analysis which will be facilitated by the ready availability of clinical data, a way of obtaining this has been suggested in this volume. However, further progress in comprehension of the underlying pathology must await a realisation of the need to increase the basic science input into male reproductive physiology.

INDEX

117

sperm production deficiencies, causes 16-19
sperm reservoirs
  high vasal blocks 40, 41
  implantable 40, 41
sperm washing, antisperm antibodies 64
sperm-zona interaction 103, 104
steroid therapy, antisperm antibodies 64
subfertility 81
surgery and infertility 2, 6

tamoxifen, semen effect 88
technetium-99 pertechnetate, scrotum
      scanning 49, 50
testes, lymphocyte infiltration 69
testes size 3, 22
  sperm count 22
testicular abnormalities 16-18
testicular biopsy 36, 46
testicular damage 7
testicular failure treatments 86
testicular maldescent 7
testicular obstruction
  antisperm antibodies 62, 63
  ejaculatory tract 3
  outflow passages 31, 32
  sites 32, 44, 45
  surgical treatments 44, 45
  surgery 41-5
  unilateral 44, 45
    causes and sites 44, 45
    treatment and pregnancy 44
testicular volume and varicocele treatment
      success 52, 54
testosterone undecanoate 87
thermography, contact for varicocele 50
Timed Exposure Photomicrography 71
transcatheterization 52, 53, 56
  complication risk 56
tray agglutination test (TAT) 60
  assessment, antisperm antibodies 74
  procedure 76
treatment
  computer data 8
  infertile male 18, 19
Trichomonas vaginalis mycoplasmas 93
tube-slide agglutination test assessment,
    antisperm antibodies 74

uro-genital examination 9

varicocele 49-57
  adolescents 49
    prophylactic treatment 56, 57
  aetiology 49
  detection 3, 4
  deterioration 57
  diagnosis 50, 51
  effects of 49
  fertility assessment 52

incidence 49, 54
incidentally discovered, approach 56
infertility risk 49, 56
pathological mechanisms 49, 50
scrotal skin temperature 50
stage and treatment success 54
subclinical 50
transcatheter embolization 52, 53, 56
  tissue adhesive 53
treatment 7, 52
  evaluation 53
  success 52-4
varicocoelectomy 18
Varioscreen 50
vas
  absent 32, 36, 46
    surgical reconstruction 36
  blocked 32
    causes 35, 36
    sperm reservoir 40, 41
    testicular obstruction 44
    treatment 39
    vasectomy reversal 43
  unilateral absence 46
vasectomy 35
  antisperm antibodies 62, 63
  reversal 38, 42, 43
    antisperm antibodies 62, 63
    comparisons 42
    factors affecting success 42
    failure, causes 42
    pregnancies 43
    re-exploration 43

vasogram
  causa epididymis 34
  ejaculatory duct cyst 39
  normal 37
vasography 36
  procedure 37
vaso-vasostomy 38, 39
  anastomosis 39
  pregnancy interval 47
venography, retrograde, spermatic vein
reflux 51
video analysis systems 100

white blood cells
  accessory gland infection 95
  prostatic fluid 91
  semen 92, 94, 95

Young's syndrome 1, 5, 32
  aetiology 34
  cilia 47
  epididymis block 33, 41

zona-free hamster eggs, penetration and
    fertility 104, 105, 107